T0297650

MIGS
Advances in Glaucoma Surgery

MIGS
Advances in Glaucoma Surgery

Edited by

Malik Y. Kahook, MD
The Slater Family Endowed Chair in Ophthalmology
Professor of Ophthalmology
Director of Clinical and Translational Research
Chief, Glaucoma Service at the University of Colorado Eye Center
University of Colorado School of Medicine
Aurora, Colorado

Associate Editors

Sarwat Salim, MD, FACS
Associate Professor of Ophthalmology
Director, Glaucoma Service
Hamilton Eye Institute
University of Tennessee
Memphis, Tennessee

Leonard K. Seibold, MD
Assistant Professor of Ophthalmology
University of Colorado Eye Center
University of Colorado School of Medicine
Aurora, Colorado

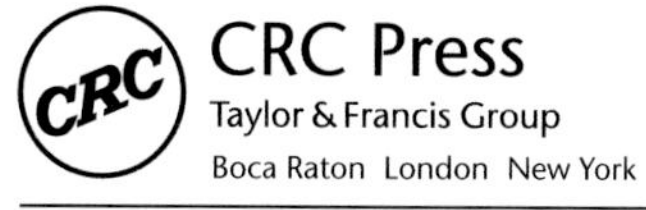

CRC Press is an imprint of the
Taylor & Francis Group, an **informa** business

Top left figure reprinted with permission from Glaukos Corporation; middle left figure reprinted with permission from Ivantis Inc; and bottom left figure reprinted with permission from Transcend Medical, Inc (Menlo Park, CA).

First published 2014 by SLACK Incorporated

Published 2024 by CRC Press
2385 NW Executive Center Drive, Suite 320, Boca Raton FL 33431

and by CRC Press
4 Park Square, Milton Park, Abingdon, Oxon, OX14 4RN

CRC Press is an imprint of Taylor & Francis Group, LLC

Library of Congress Cataloging-in-Publication Data

MIGS : advances in glaucoma surgery / edited by Malik Y. Kahook ; associate editors, Sarwat Salim, Leonard K. Seibold.
p. ; cm.
Minimally invasive glaucoma surgery
Advances in glaucoma surgery
Includes bibliographical references and index.
ISBN 978-1-61711-600-1 (paperback : alk. paper)
I. Kahook, Malik Y., editor of compilation. II. Salim, Sarwat, editor of compilation. III. Seibold, Leonard K., editor of compilation. IV. Title: Minimally invasive glaucoma surgery. V. Title: Advances in glaucoma surgery.
[DNLM: 1. Glaucoma--surgery. 2. Ophthalmologic Surgical Procedures--methods. 3. Surgical Procedures, Minimally Invasive--methods. WW 290]
RE871
617.7'41--dc23
2013026985

ISBN: 9781617116001 (pbk)
ISBN: 9781003525080 (ebk)

DOI: 10.1201/9781003525080

Dedication

We dedicate this book to our families for their constant support and generous encouragement.

Contents

About the Editor

Malik Y. Kahook, MD, is Professor of Ophthalmology and The Slater Family Endowed Chair in Ophthalmology at the University of Colorado School of Medicine. He is Director of Clinical and Translational Research and serves as chief of the glaucoma service and director of the glaucoma fellowship at the University of Colorado Eye Center. He specializes in the medical and surgical treatment of glaucoma and cataracts. Dr. Kahook is active within the ophthalmology community including memberships in the American Academy of Ophthalmology, American Glaucoma Society, American Society of Refractive and Cataract Surgeons, and the Association for Research in Vision and Ophthalmology. He serves on the American Academy of Ophthalmology Glaucoma Committee and is a member of the American Glaucoma Society Program Committee.

Dr. Kahook has authored over 210 peer-reviewed manuscripts, abstracts, and book chapters, and is editor of *Essentials of Glaucoma Surgery* and the seminal textbook of glaucoma *Chandler and Grant's Glaucoma.* His research accomplishments are focused on multiple unmet needs including advanced cataract surgery devices and implants, treatment of macular degeneration, novel glaucoma therapies, and advanced imaging techniques. He was awarded an AGS Clinician-Scientist Fellowship Award in 2007 as well as the AGS Compliance Grant in 2006 and was named New Inventor of the Year for the University of Colorado in 2009 and Inventor of the Year for 2010. He received the American Academy of Ophthalmology Achievement Award in 2011 and the Ludwig Von Sallmann Clinician-Scientist Award (ARVO) in 2013. Dr. Kahook has filed for 12 patents, several of which have been licensed by companies for development and commercialization. He serves on several editorial boards including the *American Journal of Ophthalmology* and *International Glaucoma Review.* Dr. Kahook is a consultant to the Food and Drug Administration's Ophthalmic Device Division.

After graduating from Northeastern Ohio University's College of Medicine, Dr. Kahook completed his residency training at the University of Colorado, Rocky Mountain Lions Eye Institute in Denver, Colorado, where he was named Chief Resident. He then went on to complete a fellowship in glaucoma with Joel S. Schuman and Robert J. Noecker at the University of Pittsburgh Medical Center in Pittsburgh, Pennsylvania.

About the Associate Editors

Sarwat Salim, MD, FACS, graduated summa cum laude from the combined BA/MD program at the State University of New York. She completed her residency in ophthalmology at the State University of New York Health Science Center at Brooklyn where she was also selected by her peers and the faculty to be the Administrative Chief Resident. After residency, she completed a glaucoma fellowship at Yale University School of Medicine. Dr. Salim has served on the faculty of the Massachusetts Eye and Ear Infirmary, Harvard Medical School, and Yale University School of Medicine.

Currently, Dr. Salim is an Associate Professor of Ophthalmology and Director of Glaucoma Service at the University of Tennessee Health Science Center in Memphis, Tennessee. Dr. Salim is a Diplomate of the American Board of Ophthalmology and a Fellow of the American Academy of Ophthalmology (AAO), American Glaucoma Society, and American College of Surgeons. She serves on the Board of Directors of the Tennessee Academy of Ophthalmology and Women in Ophthalmology. She is actively involved with AAO educational and leadership initiatives and has been recognized by the Academy with both an Achievement Award and the Secretariat Award.

Dr. Salim regularly contributes to her field through her writing, research, lectures, and international outreach work. She has served as a scientific program chair for many local, national, and international meetings and has been a recipient of several awards for her leadership. Dr. Salim is a dedicated educator and mentor and has trained many local and international glaucoma fellows. She is recognized as one of the Best Doctors in America and America's Top Ophthalmologists (Consumer Research Council of America).

Leonard K. Seibold, MD, is Assistant Professor of Ophthalmology in the Department of Ophthalmology at the University of Colorado School of Medicine. He is a member of the glaucoma service and a preceptor for the glaucoma fellowship. Dr. Seibold specializes in the medical and surgical treatment of glaucoma and cataracts.

Dr. Seibold is a native of Lawton, Oklahoma and completed his undergraduate degree in 2003 from Southwestern Oklahoma State University. He then graduated from the University of Oklahoma College of Medicine in 2007, where he also completed an internship in internal medicine in 2008. He then went on to finish ophthalmology residency training in 2011 at the University of Colorado, where he also completed a fellowship in glaucoma in 2012.

He is an active member of the ophthalmology community, holding memberships with the American Academy of Ophthalmology, American Glaucoma Society, Chandler-Grant Glaucoma Society, and the Colorado Society of Eye Physicians and Surgeons. Dr. Seibold has authored over 40 peer-reviewed manuscripts, abstracts, and book chapters. He provides editorial services for numerous journals and is a member of the editorial board for the *Journal of Current Glaucoma Practice* and the *International Journal of Ophthalmology.* He currently serves on the Board of Admissions for the University of Colorado School of Medicine as well as the Board of Directors for the Colorado Society of Eye Physicians and Surgeons.

Contributing Authors

Iqbal Ike Ahmed, MD (Chapter 2)
Assistant Professor of Ophthalmology
University of Toronto
Credit Valley Eyecare
Toronto, Ontario, Canada

John P. Berdahl, MD (Chapter 10)
Cataract, Refractive, Glaucoma and Corneal Surgeon
Vance Thompson Vision
Sioux Falls, South Dakota

Jacob W. Brubaker, MD (Chapter 9)
Glaucoma and Anterior Segment Surgery
Private Practice
Sacramento, California

Sean Ianchulev, MD, MPH (Chapter 12)
Associate Clinical Professor
University of California, San Francisco
San Francisco, California

Sabita M. Ittoop, MD (Chapter 4)
Instructor, Glaucoma Fellow
Department of Ophthalmology
University of Colorado Denver
Aurora, Colorado

Ananda Kalevar, MD (Chapter 2)
Resident in Ophthalmology
McGill University
Montreal, Quebec, Canada

Mahmoud Khaimi, MD (Chapter 9)
Clinical Associate Professor of Ophthalmology
Dean McGee Eye Institute
The University of Oklahoma College of Medicine
Oklahoma City, Oklahoma

Mina B. Pantcheva, MD (Chapter 8)
Assistant Professor of Ophthalmology
University of Colorado School of Medicine
Department of Ophthalmology
Aurora, Colorado

Hady Saheb, MD, MPH (Chapter 2)
Assistant Professor of Ophthalmology
McGill University
Montreal, Quebec, Canada

Thomas W. Samuelson, MD (Chapter 5)
Glaucoma and Anterior Surgery
Minnesota Eye Consultants
Adjunct Professor
University of Minnesota
Minneapolis, Minnesota

Andrew Schieber, MSME (Chapter 5)
Senior Research and Development Engineer
Ivantis Inc
Irvine, California

Kuldev Singh, MD, MPH (Chapter 5)
Professor of Ophthalmology
Director, Glaucoma Service
Stanford University School of Medicine
Stanford, California

Jeffrey R. SooHoo, MD (Chapter 3)
Instructor/Fellow
University of Colorado School of Medicine
Department of Ophthalmology
Aurora, Colorado

Carol B. Toris, PhD (Chapter 5)
Department of Ophthalmology and Visual Sciences
University of Nebraska Medical Center
Omaha, Nebraska

Rohit Varma, MD (Chapter 7)
Professor and Chair
Illinois Eye and Ear Infirmary
UIC Department of Ophthalmology and Visual Sciences
Associate Dean for Strategic Planning
UIC College of Medicine
Chicago, Illinois

Introduction

MIGS: Advances in Glaucoma Surgery started as an exercise among colleagues to define the most exciting aspects of new innovations in glaucoma surgery. The use of minimally invasive and microincisional techniques to address intraocular pressure control was the center of the discussion and eventually the focus of this text. Many of these procedures were born out of the desire to surgically treat glaucoma without the common intraoperative and postoperative complications that are experienced with conventional filtration surgery. An ideal intervention for uncontrolled glaucoma would result in restoration of the natural outflow system with low potential for adverse events. The definition of the acronym *MIGS* has changed over time. I first heard of the acronym from Ike Ahmed, MD in 2010 and at the time it stood for "minimally invasive glaucoma surgery." The term was useful in facilitating communication between physicians and allowed for brainstorming regarding what constituted a MIGS procedure. Over time, MIGS evolved into "microincisional glaucoma surgery" so as to better characterize the sophisticated surgical approach without minimizing the skill and time needed for effective outcomes by use of the word *minimally*. We intentionally use the acronym MIGS rather than spelling out the words throughout the text as we still lack true consensus on what it stands for today. Two of our contributors explain in Chapter 2 the evolution of defining MIGS and we find their thoughts to be compelling and worthy of attention.

As with any new field in surgery, there have been some growing pains in development and regulatory approval. The new concepts introduced by the MIGS approaches required intense communication with the FDA and with the community of glaucoma experts to define proper clinical trials and endpoints. The Trabecular Micro-Bypass stent (iStent, Glaukos Corporation, Laguna Hills, CA) was approved in 2012 and has now ushered in a new era in the surgical treatment of glaucoma. Many more MIGS devices, including the Hydrus Microstent (Ivantis Inc, Irvine, CA) and the CyPass Micro-Stent (Transcend Medical, Menlo Park, CA), are in the pipeline and data are forthcoming regarding their efficacy and potential role in surgical practice. In this text, we focus on each device and unique approach that we believe belong in the MIGS category. Each chapter is designed to be self-contained as a standalone resource for the reader. We include an introductory chapter on the history of glaucoma surgery to set the stage for how MIGS fits in with previously introduced concepts and techniques. The final 2 chapters focus on emerging techniques that could be of use in the future, as well as non-MIGS procedures that might be the focus of future editions of this text.

It is our sincere hope that this text will be enjoyable to read and educational for those seeking to expand their knowledge about MIGS. We also hope it will lead to debates about the efficacy of this category of glaucoma surgery as well as the potential benefits and limitations compared to more traditional surgical procedures. The authors of each chapter worked diligently to present the information on each device. It is now up to the reader to decide if MIGS will have a lasting place in the surgical decision-making algorithm and how this field might evolve over time.

Malik Y. Kahook, MD

1

The History of Glaucoma Surgery

Leonard K. Seibold, MD

Over the past century, the management of glaucoma has broadened to include several new classes of topical medications, noninvasive laser treatments, and incisional surgery. Despite the expansion of treatment options, the objective of all therapeutic modalities continues to focus solely on the reduction of intraocular pressure (IOP). Physicians must now consider all of the available options before determining the treatment plan best suited for each particular patient. Topical medications for glaucoma have not only grown in number, but also offer improved efficacy of IOP lowering and tolerability to patients with less frequent dosing. The development and improvement of laser trabeculoplasty has likewise drawn favor from clinicians and patients as initial treatment for its similar efficacy, one-time application, and noninvasive nature. Likewise, traditional glaucoma surgery has progressed through many iterations and modifications over the past 100 years.

Despite the evolution of traditional glaucoma surgery, the basic mechanism has been singularly focused on filtering procedures. Essentially, a filtering procedure involves the creation of a new, alternative pathway for aqueous humor to exit the eye thus bypassing the natural outflow system. The resultant drainage fistula allows aqueous to avoid the trabecular meshwork, Schlemm's canal, and the downstream collector channels. With this general principle in mind, glaucoma surgeons have strived to modify and advance surgical technique to achieve consistent and durable IOP reduction while reducing complications and adverse outcomes for patients. The quest to restore the natural aqueous outflow system rather than bypassing it has remained a central goal for new surgical procedures. The introduction of minimally invasive glaucoma procedures is a step toward realizing this goal.

Full-Thickness Filtering Surgery

Albrecht von Graefe is credited for performing the first glaucoma surgery in 1856 when he discovered that an iridectomy could be therapeutic in cases of angle closure and several secondary glaucomas (Figure 1-1).[1] Two years later, Louis De Wecker introduced the initial iteration of filtering surgery with the full-thickness anterior sclerotomy. His procedure involved the creation of a full-thickness scleral incision 1 mm posterior to the limbus with an overlying conjunctival flap that resulted in a filtration cicatrix through which intraocular fluid may exit the eye (Figure 1-2).[1]

Kahook MY.
MIGS: Advances in Glaucoma Surgery (pp 1-11).

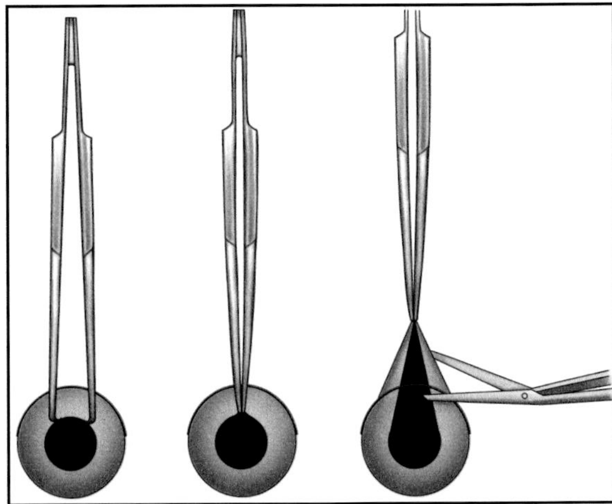

Figure 1-1. Iridectomy. After a large superior limbal incision is made, iris forceps are used to grasp the iris near the pupillary margin. The iris is retracted out of the wound and cut with scissors.

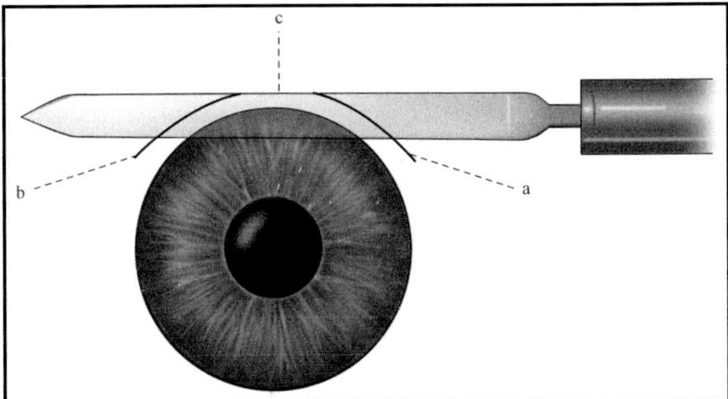

Figure 1-2. Anterior sclerotomy. A von Graefe cataract knife is introduced 1 mm from the limbus at point (a) and advanced across the anterior chamber to emerge at point (b). The incision is then advanced upward to enlarge the wound, leaving a narrow bridge of intact sclera at point (c). The knife is tilted to permit aqueous egress and the knife is removed.

In 1871, he modified the procedure to avoid iris prolapse using miotics and careful repositioning of the iris.[2] Complications included iris prolapse, inadvertent corneal incision, anterior chamber flattening, and lens disruption.[1] Later modifications were made to avoid iris prolapse using alternate incision techniques and daily ocular massage was advocated postoperatively to improve outcomes.[3] In 1894, De Wecker further modified the procedure by combining iridodialysis at the time of anterior sclerotomy to create a new procedure.[1] However, despite several modifications, the procedure failed to produce safe, reliable, long-term successful results and was largely abandoned by the early 1900s.

In 1906, LaGrange presented irido-sclerotomy as another full-thickness filtering procedure.[2] His procedure involved making a large conjunctival flap followed by a full-thickness scleracorneal incision at the limbus. An anterior piece of sclera was removed from the wound followed by an iridectomy and then closure of the conjunctiva to create the filtering cicatrix (Figure 1-3). The procedure was later modified by Holth who used punch forceps to complete the sclerectomy.[1]

In 1909, Fergus and Elliot utilized trephination as an alternative to scissors and forceps for creation of a sclerectomy.[4,5] Elliot described a small limbal incision to split the peripheral cornea allowing an anterior full-thickness trephination of sclerocorneal tissue (Figure 1-4). Sugar later advocated a more posterior sclerolimbal trephination to avoid thinner filtering blebs.[6] Although initial infection rates were low, trephination fell out of favor due to common complications of flat anterior chamber and cataract formation.

The iridencleisis operation was introduced by Sugar in 1906.[2] In this procedure, a full-thickness scleral incision is again made, but rather than avoiding iris prolapse or performing an iridectomy, iris tissue is deliberately incarcerated into the wound. As initially described, a radial iris incision was performed from the iris base to the pupil and the cut edges were then pulled into the scleral wound (Figure 1-5). This unique step was added as a means to maintain patency of the aqueous

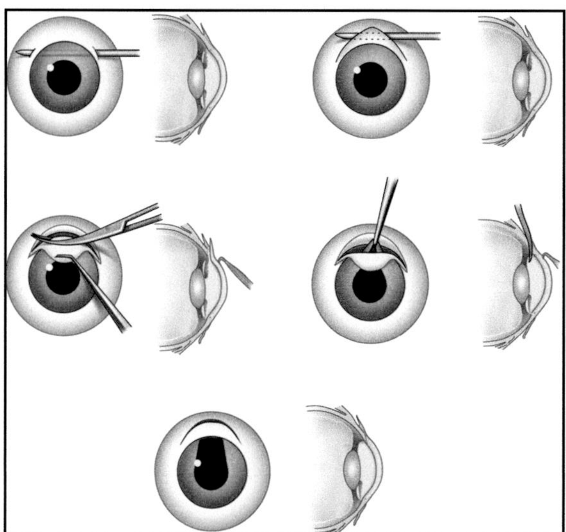

Figure 1-3. The LaGrange procedure. A narrow von Graefe knife is advanced across the anterior chamber from 1 mm outside of the limbus to a similar location at the opposite limbus. The knife is advanced and brought out superiorly to complete a conjunctival and scleral flap. The conjunctiva is held forward and the scleral flap excised followed by iridectomy. The conjunctival flap is then replaced.

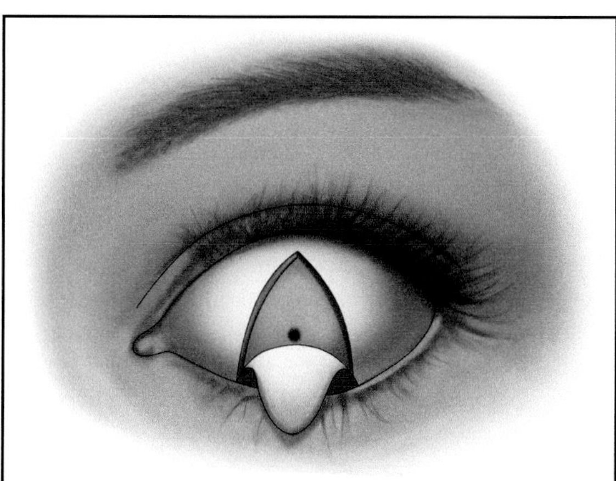

Figure 1-4. Trephination. A conjunctival flap is reflected onto the cornea and a full thickness trephination of sclerocorneal tissue is made to enter the anterior chamber. The conjunctival flap is then replaced.

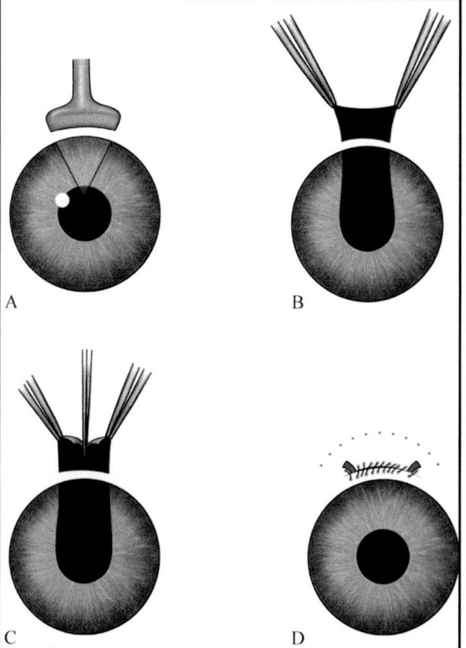

Figure 1-5. Iridencleisis. (A) After a conjunctival flap is made, a full thickness corneoscleral wound is created to enter the anterior chamber. (B) The adjacent iris is grasped at either end of the wound and externalized through the wound. (C) Scissors are used to bisect the iris into 2 pillars that are then (D) deliberately incarcerated in the wound.

outflow channel. Surgeons later abandoned this procedure due to the undesirable cosmetic effects on the iris in addition to its purported association with sympathetic ophthalmia.[7]

Later in 1924, Preziosi first described the use of electrocautery to create a limbal fistula into the anterior chamber.[8] This concept was harnessed by Scheie in 1958, when he described his technique of thermal sclerostomy.[9] The technique involves a 5-mm limbal scratch incision placed just posterior to the limbus. Cautery is then applied to the wound edges until a separation of 1 mm is achieved. The egress of aqueous would inhibit the application of cautery but later use of bipolar wet field cautery avoided this problem. Unfortunately, Scheie's operation encountered similar problems to the trephination procedure.

All of these early glaucoma surgeries were derived from the creation of a full-thickness fistula through which aqueous outflow was achieved. While initially effective, they all uniformly failed due to eventual uncontrolled scarring or resulted in serious vision-threatening complications such as hypotony, flat anterior chamber, cataract formation, and infection.[1,2] These complications were largely due to the uncontrolled nature of aqueous outflow created by each operation. While technique evolved to smaller incision size, little attempt was made to limit flow through the fistula. These significant limitations led to the next major advancement of filtering surgery in glaucoma, guarded filtration.

Guarded Filtration Surgery

The initial technique of trabeculectomy was suggested by Sugar in 1961 but popularized by Cairns in 1968.[10,11] He designed his procedure based on the assumption that the site of greatest resistance to outflow occurred at the trabecular meshwork and inner wall of Schlemm's canal. Therefore by removing a piece of trabecular meshwork and Schlemm's canal, he could create an unobstructed pathway for aqueous to exit into the exposed, cut ends of Schlemm's canal and out of the eye through aqueous veins. The initial technique involved the creation of a partial-thickness corneoscleral flap at the limbus. A portion of trabecular meshwork and Schlemm's canal was then excised and the flap sutured securely back in place. While the procedure was effective at lowering IOP, the mechanism of aqueous outflow did not appear to be through Schlemm's canal as intended. Evaluation of primate and human eyes found that cut ends of the canal underwent fibrotic closure.[12,13] Instead, external filtration around the flap edges or through the flap was found to be present in studies of eyes with successful trabeculectomies.[14] Furthermore, the presence of filtering blebs was noted in most successful outcomes, suggesting that the procedure functions predominately as a guarded external filtration surgery.[15] While the primary route of outflow appears to be around the flap edges, other proposed routes of aqueous exit include filtration through the scleral flap, flow into the cut ends of Schlemm's canal, and cyclodialysis clefts when tissue is removed posterior to the scleral spur.[12,16,17]

The modern day trabeculectomy procedure employs a similar technique of Cairns' operation, although important modifications have been made in the interim as well. In 1970, Watson began his dissection of Schlemm's canal and trabecular meshwork posteriorly for improved visualization of excised tissue.[18] More recently, surgeons make an incision into the anterior chamber beneath the scleral flap, and then use a tissue punch to remove sclerocorneal tissue from the posterior wound lip. The overlying scleral flap is then secured somewhat loosely to regulate flow through the sclerotomy (Figure 1-6). In fact, today little, if any, trabecular meshwork is removed because this is irrelevant to the creation of a guarded fistula leading to the formation of an external filtration bleb. Despite this fact, the moniker "trabeculectomy" is still used today. Other notable modifications of technique include using a fornix-based conjunctival flap, altering the shape and size of the scleral flap, postoperative lysis of scleral flap sutures, and placement of releasable flap sutures.[19]

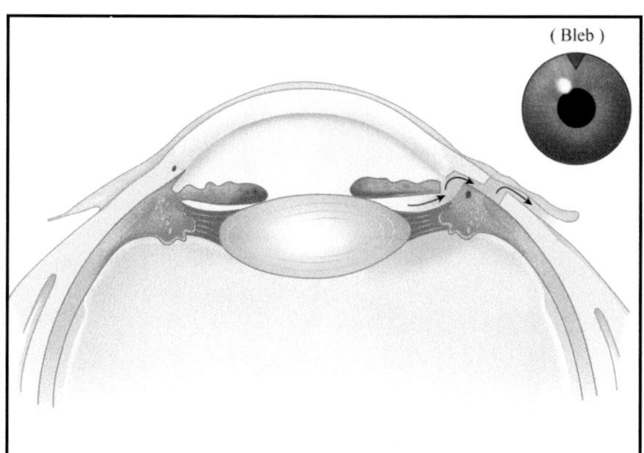

Figure 1-6. Trabeculectomy. Aqueous fluid predominantly exits the eye through an opening guarded by the overlying partial thickness flap. Fluid then accumulates in a subconjunctival bleb.

Wound Modulation

Perhaps the most profound alteration of trabeculectomy has been the introduction of antifibrotics. The evolution of filtration surgery to a guarded procedure served to significantly minimize early complications of overfiltration; however, subsequent failure and scarring of outflow pathways remained a problem. This led to the search for methods and agents capable of modulating the wound-healing process after surgery in order to prolong function of filtration blebs. In 1965, Sugar first described the beneficial effects of corticosteroids on conjunctival blebs.[20] Later studies confirmed their benefit to long-term efficacy in trabeculectomy, prompting their widespread use before, during, and after filtration surgery.[21]

In 1983, Chen et al discovered that the alkylating agent mitomycin C (MMC) used intraoperatively resulted in favorable success rates.[22] As a result of this early success, multiple later investigations of MMC found that its use decreased surgical failure rate in various glaucoma populations and helped to achieve a lower IOP.[21] Then in 1984, Gressel et al described the first use of the antimetabolite 5-fluorouracil (5-FU) as an adjunctive treatment after trabeculectomy.[23] By inhibiting nucleotide synthesis, the medication resulted in the death of fibroblasts and other cells involved in the healing process, thereby minimizing scar formation. Initially used in eyes at high risk for failure, 5-FU was injected subconjunctivally multiple times during the postoperative period. Toxicity to corneal and conjunctival epithelium later led to intraoperative application of the drug with favorable results.[21]

While antifibrotics' greatest benefit seemed to come in eyes at highest risk for failure, surgeons now routinely use them as a standard step of trabeculectomy in most settings.[24] The survival benefit of antifibrotics comes with inherent risks though. Their use has been associated with the formation of thin, cystic blebs that are susceptible to late-onset leaks and an increased risk of endophthalmitis.[25] Thus, a superior method of wound modulation is needed to make trabeculectomy a safer and more effective procedure. Several alternative methods and agents have been described, but none have achieved superior results to MMC in a large-scale prospective study.[21]

More recent attempts have been made to improve wound modulation in the hopes of maintaining or exceeding success rates of the antifibrotics while decreasing adverse effects. In 2002, CAT-152, a monoclonal antibody against transforming growth factor-beta2 (TGF-ß2), was studied as a more targeted approach to wound modulation.[26] After promising initial trials, subsequent large randomized trials in 2007 failed to show a benefit over placebo.[27-29] In 2010, Kahook found anti-vascular endothelial growth factor (VEGF) therapy to achieve more desirable bleb characteristics when compared with MMC alone.[30] In an animal model, Sherwood described that while individual targeted therapy to reduce wound healing after filtration surgery was beneficial over control, a sequential and multiple drug treatment approach provided additional efficacy benefit

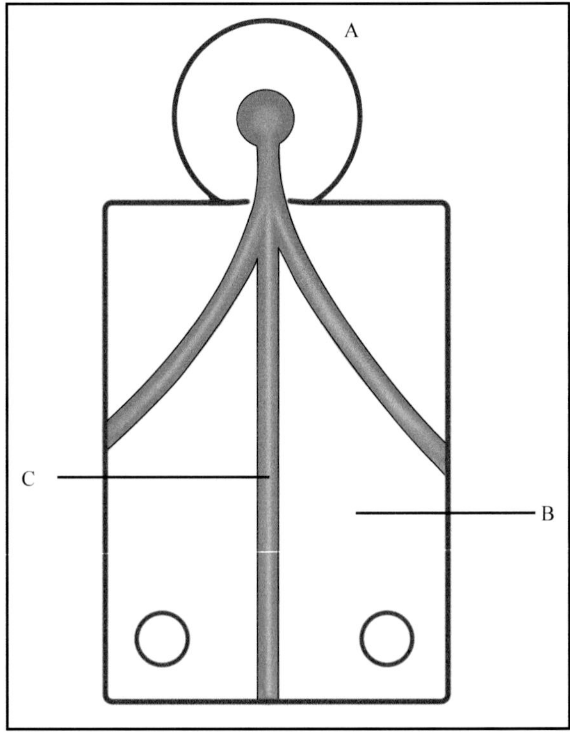

Figure 1-7. Qadeer glaucoma drainage device. The circular head (A) was inserted into the anterior chamber with the body (B) secured to sclera. Aqueous could exit along 1 of 3 drainage channels (C) to a subconjunctival bleb.

while not compromising safety.[31] Multiple other methods and agents of wound modulation have since been studied, including radiation, gene therapy, and photodynamic therapy among others.[21]

Tube Shunt Surgery

Shortly after the introduction of full-thickness filtering procedures, attempts were made to maintain a patent drainage fistula through the use of implanted materials. The earliest report of this was in 1876, when De Wecker placed a gold wire implant after failed iridectomy.[3] Later in 1906, Rollet implanted a horsehair at the limbus to bridge the tract between the anterior chamber and the subconjunctival space.[32] This was followed by multiple endeavors utilizing solid structures, or setons, as a means of preventing closure of the newly created filtering tract. Among those described are silk threads, hairs, gold, platinum, tantalum, glass, and polythene tube.[33] These efforts still failed over time due to foreign body reaction and limbal scar formation, migration of implant, and erosion through conjunctiva.

After Ridley first described the biocompatibility of plastic lenses in the eye,[34] Qadeer utilized a polymethyl methacrylate (PMMA) plate for the basis of his subconjunctival drainage device.[35] The plate was elegantly constructed with a smaller head to be inserted into the anterior chamber and a larger posterior portion engraved with drainage channels placed subconjunctivally (Figure 1-7). While the device had similar limitations of prior seton-style implants, it overcame the issue of foreign body reaction and was an early utilization of a subconjunctival plate for bleb formation. In the late 1950s, Epstein and Ellis described the use of translimbal drainage tubes to allow aqueous to exit through a hollow lumen.[36,37] Despite maintaining a patent fistula and early success at filtration, scarring and fibrosis of the bleb downstream inhibited drainage and led to systematic failure.

The modern tube shunt was first introduced by Molteno in 1969.[38] In his initial design, he utilized a similar translimbal drainage tube inserted into the anterior chamber and incorporated

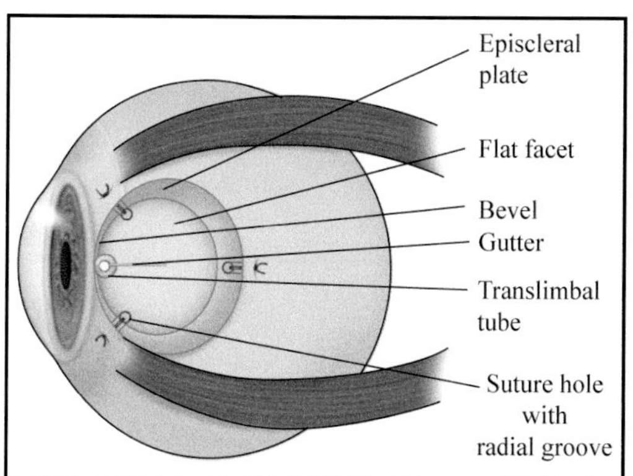

Figure 1-8. The original Molteno drainage implant.

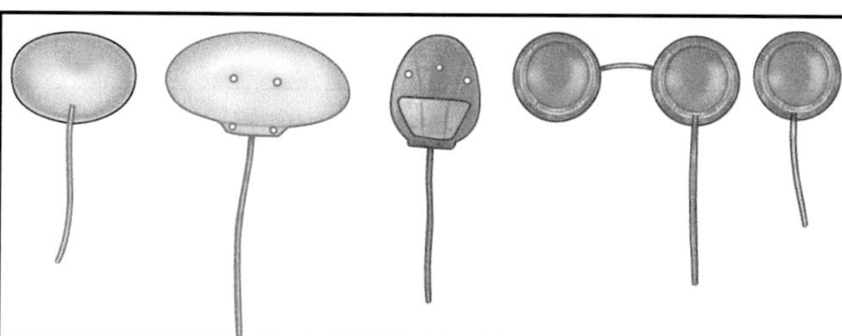

Figure 1-9. Glaucoma drainage devices. From left to right: Krupin drainage device, Baerveldt 350 mm^2 drainage implant, Ahmed valve implant, double plate Molteno device, and single plate Molteno device.

a thin external plate at the other end (Figure 1-8). The broad plate was designed to be fixated to sclera beneath Tenon's capsule and conjunctiva to maintain the aqueous reservoir and promote bleb formation. The large plate situated near the limbus resulted in large anterior blebs that caused problems such as corneal dellen, plate exposure, and dysesthesia. A few years later he modified the procedure to divert aqueous to a remote location to the limbus. He used a much longer silicone tube that could reach a large plate placed 9 to 10 mm posterior to the limbus and situated between the rectus muscles.[39] This modification became the standard format for which all modern tube shunts follow (Figure 1-9). The device was not without limitations though as aqueous could flow unrestricted, resulting in hypotony, flat anterior chambers, and choroidal effusions.[33] Therefore, unrestricted devices are ligated today with some form of temporary ligature or stent.

The next major modification to tube shunts came in 1976 when Krupin and colleagues introduced the concept of a flow-restricting valve.[40] The original design consisted of a Supramid tube sealed to an external Silastic tube with a slit valve. The unidirectional valve was designed to open at an IOP between 9 and 11 mm Hg to maintain a low but controlled pressure. The device was later modified to include an external plate like the Molteno to prevent subconjunctival fibrosis and scarring.[41] In 1993, Ahmed introduced another pressure-sensitive device involving a sheet valve housed within a polypropylene body designed to open when the pressure is between 8 and 10 mm Hg.[42] The valve feature of these devices offered the possibility of achieving predictable and controlled outflow after surgery. However, the novel component also created new valve-related complications, including valve blockage or malfunction that could result in uncontrolled IOP or hypotony.[43]

Subsequent modifications in tube shunt surgery include the enlargement of end plate surface area to achieve lower IOP. In 1981, Molteno introduced a double-plate implant composed of a standard tube and plate and a second plate connected to the first one by a separate silicone tube.[44] The Ahmed valve implant (New World Medical, Inc, Rancho Cucamonga, CA) also offers a dual-plate option for improved IOP control.[45] Instead of 2 smaller plates, Baerveldt designed an implant with a uniquely large surface area plate.[46] The plates ranged from 250 to 500 mm^2 and could be

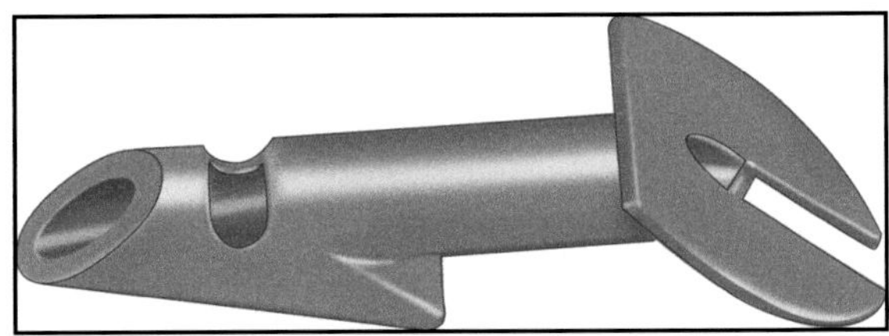

Figure 1-10. The EX-PRESS glaucoma drainage device.

placed under the rectus muscles. Despite the advantage of improved pressure control with larger or multiple plates, complications such as diplopia and hypotony also increased with these alterations.

Tube shunt surgery has historically been reserved for refractory glaucoma cases in which prior trabeculectomy has failed or in situations where traditional filtering surgery is at high risk for failure. This trend has changed significantly over recent years as surgeons have become more comfortable with proper surgical procedure and postoperative management of tube shunts. In fact, Medicare data have shown a steady reduction in trabeculectomy with a concurrent increase in tube shunt surgery.[47] Additionally, in a recent multicenter randomized trial, tube shunt surgery achieved a higher success rate compared to trabeculectomy at 5 years in eyes that had previous trabeculectomy or cataract removal.[48] Nonetheless, no consensus has been declared over which filtration surgery is superior. Importantly, neither procedure is without the risk of severe vision-threatening complications that patients could be faced with their entire lives after surgery.

EX-PRESS

The EX-PRESS glaucoma drainage device (Alcon, Fort Worth, TX) is the most recent development in full-thickness filtering surgery (Figure 1-10). The implant has acquired its own surgical classification as it does not fit the typical mold of previous tube shunts and is distinctly dissimilar from a traditional trabeculectomy. Advancements in microsurgical device manufacturing allowed the production of this stainless steel mini-shunt measuring approximately 3 mm in length and with a lumen diameter of only 50 µm.[49] The back plate of the device was designed to rest flush against the sclera while the distal end extended into the anterior chamber. However, no large external plate or long tube was present, distinguishing the EX-PRESS from other tube shunt devices.

After initial FDA approval in 2002, the device was implanted subconjunctivally near the limbus as a rapid, efficient glaucoma-filtering operation.[50] Unfortunately, flow restriction of the lumen was insufficient and many cases resulted in hypotony. In addition, the lack of overlying coverage of the device resulted in frequent conjunctival erosion. These complications prompted a revised technique in which the implant was inserted beneath a scleral flap that is secured to achieve adequate device coverage and flow restriction.[51] Despite the similarities of this technique to trabeculectomy, the currently accepted procedure does not require corneoscleral tissue removal or a peripheral iridectomy. The device removed this large variable of standard guarded filtration surgery and allowed for a more controlled and consistent outflow pathway. This has translated into a more predictable postoperative outcome with less incidence of hypotony and choroidal effusion.[52]

Nonpenetrating Glaucoma Surgery

In an attempt to avoid a penetrating wound and filtration bleb, Kraznov described his sinusotomy technique in 1968.[53] The procedure involved removal of a narrow band of sclera adjacent to Schlemm's canal across 4 clock hours. He rationalized this technique by his belief that the greatest resistance to aqueous outflow was located at the scleral aqueous veins, and not necessarily at the trabecular meshwork. Therefore, he could avoid entering the anterior chamber and leave behind an intact trabecular meshwork and inner wall of Schlemm's canal. In 1984, Zimmerman described a similar technique termed *nonpenetrating trabeculectomy* where the entirety of Schlemm's canal was removed in addition to the outer layers of trabecular meshwork, leaving the inner layers intact.[54] Later in 1990, Fyodorov and Kozlov described the technique of deep sclerectomy, still used today.[55,56] In deep sclerectomy, a second, deeper scleral flap is dissected anteriorly to unroof Schlemm's canal and then excised to create an intrascleral lake for aqueous to drain into. The inner wall of Schlemm's canal and juxtacannalicular meshwork is also removed to reveal a thin trabeculo-descemetic window through which aqueous can easily flow.

The nonpenetrating procedure was then modified further in 1999, when Stegmann published his technique for viscocanalostomy.[57] Using a similar technique to deep sclerectomy, Schlemm's canal was unroofed to expose 2 patent ends of the canal. A small cannula was then introduced into both openings of the canal and viscoelastic was gently injected to dilate the canal. The surgery was believed to augment aqueous outflow through the mechanical opening of the canal and potential inhibition of fibrosis by the viscoelastic. All of these nonpenetrating surgeries offer the potential advantage of decreased complications due to their avoidance of a full-thickness wound and risk of hypotony. Some are still in favor today in certain parts of the world; however, they have failed to replace trabeculectomy due to their relatively inadequate efficacy over time, as they are subject to subsequent scarring and failure. They do represent an important advance in surgical technique for glaucoma procedures.

The Next Step

While surgical techniques have improved over the years and incorporated the use of drainage devices, glaucoma surgery has continued to hinge on one singular concept: the creation of an alternative full-thickness drainage fistula for the drainage of aqueous from the eye. This approach has been proven effective, yet continues to be plagued with shortcomings that are still present today despite modifications and improvements over the past century. These include potentially vision-threatening complications like hypotony, wound leaks, infection, inflammation, and postoperative scarring with loss of effect over time. Thus, physicians and patients facing these risks have often delayed surgical therapy as a last resort in the glaucoma treatment paradigm. While innovation has improved outcomes, following this same vein of surgical approach has not yielded a major innovation for surgeons or patients in many years. Now, facing a substantial projected increase in glaucoma burden within the aging population, the need for a safer, more reliable surgical armamentarium has never been greater.

Finally, a new wave of glaucoma surgery is upon us: MIGS. This novel surgical genre offers new ideas of micro incisions and implants that promise to avoid pitfalls of traditional surgery. Innovators in this field have sought to exploit new avenues of IOP reduction predominantly by improving or modifying the existing, natural outflow pathways rather than abandoning them altogether. Less commonly, alternative avenues have also been taken in MIGS. These include procedures that reduce aqueous inflow or utilize ab interno approaches to establish a new yet physiologic outflow. All of these procedures offer surgeons and patients the potential for a much faster and safer glaucoma surgery that allows rapid recovery and more predictable outcomes postoperatively. Many of these can easily be combined at the time of cataract surgery as well. In addition, by minimizing potential risks, surgical options can now be approached at a much earlier stage of glaucomatous disease. While filtering surgeries have slowly evolved along the same line over the past century, MIGS now represents a paradigm shift in glaucoma therapy that has been a long time coming.

References

1. Wood CA. *A System of Ophthalmic Operations; Being a Complete Treatise on the Operative Conduct of Ocular Diseases and Some Extraocular Conditions Causing Eye Symptoms.* Chicago, IL: Cleveland Press; 1911.
2. Sugar HS. *The Glaucomas.* 2nd ed. New York, NY: Hoeber-Harper; 1957.
3. Razeghinejad MR, Spaeth GL. A history of the surgical management of glaucoma. *Optom Vis Sci.* 2011;88(1):E39-E47.
4. Elliot R. A preliminary note on a new operative procedure for the establishment of a filtering cicatrix in the treatment of glaucoma. *Ophthalmoscope.* 1909;7:804-806.
5. Fergus F. Treatment of glaucoma by trephining. *Br Med J.* 1909;2:983-984.
6. Sugar HS. Limbal trepanation: fourteen years' experience. *Ann Ophthalmol.* 1975;7:1399-1404.
7. Harris D. Sympathetic ophthalmia following iridencleisis. Case report and incidence. *Am J Ophthalmol.* 1961;51:829-831.
8. Preziosi CL. The electro-cautery in the treatment of glaucoma. *Br J Ophthalmol.* 1924;8:414-417.
9. Scheie HG. Retraction of scleral wound edges as a fistulizing procedure for glaucoma. *Trans Am Acad Ophthalmol Otolaryngol.* 1958;62:803-811.
10. Cairns JE. Trabeculectomy. Preliminary report of a new method. *Am J Ophthalmol.* 1968;66(4):673-679.
11. Sugar HS. Experimental trabeculectomy in glaucoma. *Am J Ophthalmol.* 1961;51:623-627.
12. Rich AM, McPherson SD. Trabeculectomy in the owl monkey. *Ann Ophthalmol.* 1973;5:1082-1088.
13. Spencer WH. Symposium: microsurgery of the outflow channels. Histologic evaluation of microsurgical glaucoma techniques. *Trans Am Acad Ophthalmol Otolaryngol.* 1972;76:389-397.
14. Shields MB. Trabeculectomy vs full-thickness filtering operation for control of glaucoma. *Ophthalmic Surg.* 1980;11:498-505.
15. Linnér E. Aqueous humor outflow pathways following trabeculectomy in patients with glaucoma [in German]. *Klin Monbl Augenheilkd.* 1989;195:291-293.
16. Benedikt O. The mode of action of trabeculectomy (author's transl) [in German]. *Klin Monbl Augenheilkd.* 1975;167:679-685.
17. Benedikt O. Demonstration of aqueous outflow patterns of normal and glaucomatous human eyes through the injection of fluorescein solution in the anterior chamber (author's transl) [in German]. *Albrecht Von Graefes Arch Klin Exp Ophthalmol.* 1976;199:45-67.
18. Watson P. Trabeculectomy: a modified ab externo technique. *Ann Ophthalmol.* 1970;2:199-206.
19. Razeghinejad MR, Fudemberg SJ, Spaeth GL. The changing conceptual basis of trabeculectomy: a review of past and current surgical techniques. *Surv Ophthalmol.* 2012;57:1-25.
20. Sugar HS. Clinical effect of corticosteroids on conjunctival filtering blebs; a case report. *Am J Ophthalmol.* 1965;59:854-860.
21. Seibold LK, Sherwood MB, Kahook MY. Wound modulation after filtration surgery. *Surv Ophthalmol.* 2012;57:530-550.
22. Chen CW. Enhanced intraocular pressure controlling effectiveness of trabeculectomy by local application of mitomycin-C. *Trans Asia Pac Acad Ophthalmol.* 1983;9:172-177.
23. Gressel MG, Parrish RK II, Folberg R. 5-fluorouracil and glaucoma filtering surgery: I. An animal model. *Ophthalmology.* 1984;91:378-383.
24. Joshi AB, Parrish RK II, Feuer WF. 2002 survey of the American Glaucoma Society: practice preferences for glaucoma surgery and antifibrotic use. *J Glaucoma.* 2005;14:172-174.
25. Lama PJ, Fechtner RD. Antifibrotics and wound healing in glaucoma surgery. *Surv Ophthalmol.* 2003;48:314-346.
26. Cordeiro MF, Gay JA, Khaw PT. Human anti-transforming growth factor-beta2 antibody: a new glaucoma anti-scarring agent. *Invest Ophthalmol Vis Sci.* 1999;40:2225-2234.
27. Khaw P, Grehn F, Hollo G, et al. A phase III study of subconjunctival human anti-transforming growth factor beta(2) monoclonal antibody (CAT-152) to prevent scarring after first-time trabeculectomy. *Ophthalmology.* 2007;114:1822-1830.
28. Siriwardena D, Khaw PT, King AJ, et al. Human antitransforming growth factor beta(2) monoclonal antibody--a new modulator of wound healing in trabeculectomy: a randomized placebo controlled clinical study. *Ophthalmology.* 2002;109:427-431.
29. Mead AL, Wong TT, Cordeiro MF, Anderson IK, Khaw PT. Evaluation of anti-TGF-beta2 antibody as a new postoperative anti-scarring agent in glaucoma surgery. *Invest Ophthalmol Vis Sci.* 2003;44:3394-3401.
30. Kahook MY. Bleb morphology and vascularity after trabeculectomy with intravitreal ranibizumab: a pilot study. *Am J Ophthalmol.* 2010;150:399-403.e1.
31. Sherwood MB. A sequential, multiple-treatment, targeted approach to reduce wound healing and failure of glaucoma filtration surgery in a rabbit model (an American Ophthalmological Society thesis). *Trans Am Ophthalmol Soc.* 2006;104:478-492.

32. Rollet M. Le drainage au irin de la chambre anterieure contre l'hypertonie et al douleur. *Rev Gen Ophthalmol.* 1906;25:481.
33. Hong CH, Arosemena A, Zurakowski D, Ayyala RS. Glaucoma drainage devices: a systematic literature review and current controversies. *Surv Ophthalmol.* 2005;50:48-60.
34. Ridley H. Intra-ocular acrylic lenses; a recent development in the surgery of cataract. *Br J Ophthalmol.* 1952;36:113-122.
35. Qadeer SA. Acrylic gonio-subconjunctival plates in glaucoma surgery. *Br J Ophthalmol.* 1954;38:353-356.
36. Epstein E. Fibrosing response to aqueous. Its relation to glaucoma. *Br J Ophthalmol.* 1959;43:641-647.
37. Ellis RA. Reduction of intraocular pressure using plastics in surgery. *Am J Ophthalmol.* 1960;50:733-742.
38. Molteno AC. New implant for drainage in glaucoma. Clinical trial. *Br J Ophthalmol.* 1969;53:606-615.
39. Molteno AC, Straughan JL, Ancker E. Long tube implants in the management of glaucoma. *S Afr Med J.* 1976;50:1062-1066.
40. Krupin T, Podos SM, Becker B, Newkirk JB. Valve implants in filtering surgery. *Am J Ophthalmol.* 1976;81:232-235.
41. Krupin eye valve with disk for filtration surgery. The Krupin Eye Valve Filtering Surgery Study Group. *Ophthalmology.* 1994;101:651-658.
42. Coleman AL, Hill R, Wilson MR, et al. Initial clinical experience with the Ahmed glaucoma valve implant. *Am J Ophthalmol.* 1995;120:23-31.
43. Feldman RM, el-Harazi SM, Villanueva G. Valve membrane adhesion as a cause of Ahmed glaucoma valve failure. *J Glaucoma.* 1997;6:10-612.
44. Molteno AC. The optimal design of drainage implants for glaucoma. *Trans Ophthalmol Soc N Z.* 1981;33:39-41.
45. Al-Aswad LA, Netland PA, Bellows AR, et al. Clinical experience with the double-plate Ahmed glaucoma valve. *Am J Ophthalmol.* 2006;141:390-391.
46. Lloyd MA, Baerveldt G, Heuer DK, Minckler DS, Martone JF. Initial clinical experience with the baerveldt implant in complicated glaucomas. *Ophthalmology.* 1994;101:640-650.
47. Ramulu PY, Corcoran KJ, Corcoran SL, Robin AL. Utilization of various glaucoma surgeries and procedures in Medicare beneficiaries from 1995 to 2004. *Ophthalmology.* 2007;114:2265-2270.
48. Gedde SJ, Schiffman JC, Feuer WJ, Herndon LW, Brandt JD, Budenz DL. Treatment outcomes in the Tube Versus Trabeculectomy (TVT) study after five years of follow-up. *Am J Ophthalmol.* 2012;153:789-803.e2.
49. Nyska A, Glovinsky Y, Belkin M, Epstein Y. Biocompatibility of the Ex-Press miniature glaucoma drainage implant. *J Glaucoma.* 2003;12:275-280.
50. Hendrick AM, Kahook MY. Ex-Press mini glaucoma shunt: surgical technique and review of clinical experience. *Expert Rev Med Devices.* 2008;5:673-677.
51. Dahan E, Carmichael TR. Implantation of a miniature glaucoma device under a scleral flap. *J Glaucoma.* 2005;14:98-102.
52. Maris PJ Jr, Ishida K, Netland PA. Comparison of trabeculectomy with Ex-Press miniature glaucoma device implanted under scleral flap. *J Glaucoma.*2007;16:14-19.
53. Krasnov MM. Externalization of Schlemm's canal (sinusotomy) in glaucoma. *Br J Ophthalmol.* 1968;52:157-161.
54. Zimmerman TJ, Kooner KS, Ford VJ, et al. Effectiveness of nonpenetrating trabeculectomy in aphakic patients with glaucoma. *Ophthalmic Surg.* 1984;15:44-50.
55. Fyodorov SN, Koslov VI, Timoshkina NT, et al. Nonpenetrating deep sclerectomy in open angle glaucoma. *Ophthalm Surg.* 1990;3:52-55.
56. Kozlov VI, Bagrov SN, Anisimova SY, et al. Nonpenetrating deep sclerectomy with collagen. *Eye Microsurgery.* 1990;3:44-46.
57. Stegmann R, Pienaar A, Miller D. Viscocanalostomy for open-angle glaucoma in black African patients. *J Cataract Refract Surg.* 1999;25:316-322.

2

What Is MIGS?

Hady Saheb, MD, MPH; Ananda Kalevar, MD; and Iqbal Ike Ahmed, MD

Trabeculectomy and glaucoma drainage device implantation remain the most commonly performed surgical procedures for the treatment of open-angle glaucoma (OAG), both being incisional ab externo surgeries. Numerous studies have shown good efficacy for these surgical procedures[1-5]; however, a high rate of complications (Tables 2-1 and 2-2)[6] has prompted the glaucoma community to search for alternative surgeries to treat OAG.

The term *MIGS* was coined by Iqbal Ike Ahmed, MD, and its definition has varied over time. The importance of defining this term has increased as more surgical options have become available, and the glaucoma treatment algorithm has evolved. In this chapter, we will define the current list of qualities and explain the advantages of the preferred description. MIGS has been described as microinvasive glaucoma surgery and minimally invasive glaucoma surgery. Microinvasiveness goes beyond the incision size of these procedures. The term *microinvasive* refers to a group of procedures that minimize the level of invasiveness and share a number of common features without minimizing the complexity of the skills to perform and develop this kind of surgery.

The importance of defining MIGS lies in the ability of a definition to frame a list of procedures with recognizable qualities. This framework facilitates the development of MIGS' role within the glaucoma treatment algorithm, the design of comparative research studies, and regulatory and commercial affairs. MIGS refers to a group of surgical procedures that share a few preferable qualities.[7]

The first is its ab interno microincisional approach. Ab interno glaucoma surgery through a clear corneal incision spares the conjunctiva of incisions and scarring. The conjunctiva-sparing approach allows the glaucoma surgeon to perform future conjunctival surgery if needed, without compromising its outcome.[8] This approach also allows direct visualization of anatomic landmarks to optimize placement of a device or incision within the angle and is easily combined with cataract surgery. Furthermore, a microincision facilitates the intraoperative maintenance of the anterior chamber and retention of normal ocular anatomy, minimizes changes in refractive outcome, and adds to procedural safety. Some ab externo surgeries such as canaloplasty, deep sclerectomy, and EX-PRESS shunt surgery have been previously included in the MIGS category. Although these procedures may offer an improved safety profile compared to trabeculectomy and tube shunt surgery,[9-11] the conjunctival incision will likely impact the outcomes of future glaucoma surgery

Kahook MY.
MIGS: Advances in Glaucoma Surgery (pp 13-16).

Table 2-1.

Early Postoperative Complications in the Tube Versus Trabeculectomy Study		
	TUBE GROUP (N = 107)	TRABECULECTOMY GROUP (N = 105)
Choroidal effusion	15(14)	14(13)
Shallow or flat anterior chamber	11(10)	10(10)
Wound leak	1(1)	12(11)
Hyphema	2(2)	8(8)
Aqueous misdirection	3(3)	1(1)
Suprachoroidal hemorrhage	2(2)	3(3)
Vitreous hemorrhage	1(1)	1(1)
Decompression retinopathy	0	1(1)
Cystoid macular edema	0	1(1)
Total number of patients with early postoperative complications	22(21)	39(37)

Reprinted with permission from Gedde SJ, Herndon LW, Brandt JD, et al. Postoperative complications in the Tube Versus Trabeculectomy (TVT) study during five years of follow-up. *Am J Ophthalmol.* 2012;153(5):804-814.e1.

Table 2-2.

Late Postoperative Complications in the Tube Versus Trabeculectomy Study		
	TUBE GROUP (N = 107)	TRABECULECTOMY GROUP (N = 105)
Persistent corneal edema	17(16)	9(9)
Dysesthesia	1(1)	8(8)
Persistent diplopia	6(6)	2(2)
Bleb leak	0	6(6)
Choroidal effusion	2(2)	4(4)
Cystoid macular edema	5(5)	2(2)
Hypotony maculopathy	1(1)	5(5)
Tube erosion	5(5)	—
Endophthalmitis/blebitis	1(1)	5(5)
Chronic or recurrent iritis	2(2)	1(1)
Tube obstruction	3(3)	—
Retinal detachment	1(1)	1(1)
Corneal ulcer	0	1(1)
Shallow or flat anterior chamber	1(1)	0
Total number of patients with late postoperative complications	36(34)	38(36)

Reprinted with permission from Gedde SJ, Herndon LW, Brandt JD, et al. Postoperative complications in the Tube Versus Trabeculectomy (TVT) study during five years of follow-up. *Am J Ophthalmol.* 2012;153(5):804-814.e1.

and may alter further surgical options. This impact on the glaucoma treatment algorithm in these patients is not consistent with one of the fundamental qualities of MIGS.

A second feature is a procedure that is minimally traumatic to the target tissue. An atraumatic approach minimizes inflammation, accelerates postoperative recovery, and maintains anatomy and physiologic outflow pathways. This approach allows the outflow resistance of the physiologic outflow pathways to prevent hypotony-related complications that are more common with surgeries that bypass the physiologic pathways. Devices in this category should also exhibit excellent biocompatibility and ideally enhance physiologic outflow pathways.

A third feature is the procedure's efficacy, which should at least be modest. Efficacy, along with the safety profile, will ultimately determine the role of these procedures within the glaucoma treatment algorithm. Proof and quantification of efficacy require randomized clinical trials. Comparative treatment arms to MIGS procedures have ranged from medications to phacoemulsification to invasive glaucoma surgeries. The most appropriate choice for the comparative study arm in MIGS studies should be the type of intervention closest to its expected role within the glaucoma treatment algorithm. This choice of intervention should also parallel the expected efficacy and safety profile of these surgeries. The efficacy of most MIGS procedures is often modest compared to more invasive glaucoma surgeries, such as trabeculectomy with mitomycin C or glaucoma drainage devices. However, this compromise in efficacy is balanced by an ultra-low risk profile.

The fourth and highly important feature of MIGS is its extremely high safety profile. These surgeries must avoid serious complications seen with other ab externo glaucoma surgeries, including hypotony, choroidal effusions, suprachoroidal hemorrhage, anterior chamber shallowing, corneal decompensation, cataract formation, diplopia, and bleb-related complications, such as bleb dysesthesia and endophthalmitis. This high safety profile allows MIGS to have an earlier role in the glaucoma treatment algorithm than more invasive surgeries.

The fifth feature is a rapid recovery with minimal impact on the patient's quality of life. Rapidity and ease of use are important features of MIGS as well, as both glaucoma specialists and comprehensive ophthalmologists should be able to perform such surgeries with a relatively short learning curve. MIGS approaches should be reasonably straightforward and may also be easily incorporated into other procedures such as cataract surgery.

The indications for MIGS are different than those for a trabeculectomy or a glaucoma drainage device. As the studies have shown modest reductions in intraocular pressure (IOP),[12-15] currently MIGS would be most suitable for patients with mild to moderate glaucoma damage and modest targeted IOP reductions. The ideal timing for a MIGS intervention continues to be clarified as we learn more about the efficacy and safety of these procedures. Given its efficacy and high safety profile, these surgeries can be considered earlier on in the glaucoma treatment algorithm than more invasive glaucoma surgeries. Combining MIGS with cataract surgery is currently the most common indication as risks of an intraocular procedure are already assumed and this combined surgery has been best studied. Indications for MIGS in the absence of cataract surgery remain to be determined as quantification of effect through randomized clinical trials is not available.

Important factors when considering MIGS include the stage of disease, the target IOP, tolerance to medications, preoperative IOP control, and the status of the angle. Patients with advanced glaucoma or those with normal tension glaucoma might require a target IOP lower than can be expected with MIGS. As MIGS enhances the physiologic outflow system rather than bypasses it, the postoperative IOP is rarely below the episcleral venous pressure. Some tolerance to medications is useful as patients can develop postoperative pressure rise due to steroid response and can temporarily require hypotensive medications. Preoperative IOP control is also important as patients with significantly uncontrolled pressure despite multiple hypotensive medications likely have diseased outflow systems refractory to MIGS. The status of the angle is also crucial in the preoperative assessment. Although combining MIGS with phacoemulsification allows a postoperative opening of the angle, patients with narrow angles may remain predisposed to peripheral anterior synechiae.

The future of MIGS is exciting. Proof and quantification of effect through well-designed randomized clinical trials should determine its evolving role in the glaucoma treatment algorithm. The authors believe that the role of MIGS will continue to evolve into an important role between medications, laser therapy, and more invasive glaucoma surgery. We may be able to treat glaucoma at an earlier stage to prevent or delay the need for more invasive surgery and its associated high risk of complications. MIGS certainly has a role within the glaucoma treatment algorithm that will likely increase and continues to be clarified.

References

1. Landers J, Martin K, Sarkies N, Bourne R, Watson P. A twenty-year follow-up study of trabeculectomy: risk factors and outcomes. *Ophthalmology.* 2012;119(4):694–702.
2. Gedde SJ, Schiffman JC, Feuer WJ, et al. Treatment outcomes in the Tube Versus Trabeculectomy (TVT) study after five years of follow-up. *Am J Ophthalmol.* 2012;153(5):789–803.e2.
3. AGIS Investigators. The Advanced Glaucoma Intervention Study (AGIS): 9. Comparison of glaucoma outcomes in black and white patients within treatment groups. *Am J Ophthalmol.* 2001;132(3):311–320.
4. Christakis PG, Kalenak JW, Zurakowski D, et al. The Ahmed Versus Baerveldt study: one-year treatment outcomes. *Ophthalmology.* 2011;118(11):2180–2189.
5. Budenz DL, Barton K, Feuer WJ, et al. Treatment outcomes in the Ahmed Baerveldt Comparison Study after 1 year of follow-up. *Ophthalmology.* 2011;118(3):443–452.
6. Gedde SJ, Herndon LW, Brandt JD, et al. Postoperative complications in the Tube Versus Trabeculectomy (TVT) study during five years of follow-up. *Am J Ophthalmol.* 2012;153(5): 804–814.e1.
7. Saheb H, Ahmed II. Micro-invasive glaucoma surgery: current perspectives and future directions. *Curr Opin Ophthalmol.* 2012;23(2):96–104.
8. Jea SY, Mosaed S, Vold SD, Rhee DJ. Effect of a failed trabectome on subsequent trabeculectomy. *J Glaucoma.* 2012;21(2):71-75.
9. Grieshaber MC, Pienaar A, Olivier J, Stegmann R. Canaloplasty for primary open-angle glaucoma: long-term outcome. *Br J Ophthalmol.* 2010;94(11):1478–1482.
10. Lewis RA, von Wolff K, Tetz M, et al. Canaloplasty: circumferential viscodilation and tensioning of Schlemm canal using a flexible microcatheter for the treatment of open-angle glaucoma in adults: two-year interim clinical study results. *J Cataract Refract Surg.* 2009;35(5):814–824.
11. Mesci C, Erbil HH, Karakurt Y, Akçakaya AA. Deep sclerectomy augmented with combination of absorbable biosynthetic sodium hyaluronate scleral implant and mitomycin-C or with mitomycin-C versus trabeculectomy: long term results. *Clin Experiment Ophthalmol.* 2011;40(4):e197-e207.
12. Arriola-Villalobos P, Martínez-de-la-Casa JM, Díaz-Valle D, Fernández-Pérez C, García-Sánchez J, García-Feijoó J. Combined iStent trabecular micro-bypass stent implantation and phacoemulsification for coexistent open-angle glaucoma and cataract: a long-term study. *Br J Ophthalmol.* 2012;96(5):645–649.
13. Samuelson TW, Katz LJ, Wells JM, Duh YJ, Giamporcaro JE; US iStent Study Group. Randomized evaluation of the trabecular micro-bypass stent with phacoemulsification in patients with glaucoma and cataract. *Ophthalmology.* 2011;118(3):459–467.
14. Craven ER, Katz LJ, Wells JM, Giamporcaro JE; iStent Study Group. Cataract surgery with trabecular micro-bypass stent implantation in patients with mild-to-moderate open-angle glaucoma and cataract: two-year follow-up. *J Cataract Refract Surg.* 2012;38(8):1339–1345.
15. Minckler D, Baerveldt G, Ramirez MA, et al. Clinical results with the Trabectome, a novel surgical device for treatment of open-angle glaucoma. *Trans Am Ophthalmol Soc.* 2006;104:40–50.

3

Basic Anatomy and Wound-Healing Considerations for MIGS

Jeffrey R. SooHoo, MD; Malik Y. Kahook, MD; and Leonard K. Seibold, MD

The success of any surgery depends upon a detailed knowledge and understanding of the relevant anatomy. Surgery to decrease intraocular pressure (IOP) in patients with glaucoma requires an intimate knowledge of the anterior segment. This becomes even more relevant when discussing newer techniques used in MIGS. Many MIGS procedures require device placement in a tissue plane with which surgeons may have little prior experience, such as Schlemm's canal (SC) or the suprachoroidal space. Gonioscopy in particular plays a central role in the intraoperative approach to these spaces and presents specific challenges that will need to be mastered to achieve enhanced outcomes. This chapter serves as a general review of anterior segment anatomy and offers pearls for practice that can be utilized in the operating room in a practical and unobtrusive manner.

Surgical Anatomy of the External Eye

Although most MIGS procedures are concerned with identification and manipulation of internal structures, it is imperative to have a firm understanding of external landmarks for appropriate wound construction in order to gain access to the anterior chamber in a safe and controlled fashion.

Limbus

In the broadest of terms, the limbus is the transition zone between the cornea and sclera. It is an important landmark in ophthalmic surgery and can be subdivided into the surgical limbus and the anatomical limbus. Anteriorly, the surgical limbus begins with the termination of clear cornea and ends posteriorly where clear cornea inserts into the sclera. The anatomical limbus is a histologic designation that refers to the termination of Descemet's membrane and Bowman's layer. When a scleral flap is created, the transition between cornea and sclera at the limbus can be identified by a grey/blue tint.

The limbus is slightly wider in the vertical meridians and may be confounded by corneal arcus or pannus frequently found superiorly. The relationship of the extraocular muscle insertions to the limbus should also be noted. The spiral of Tillaux describes this relationship, with the medial

Kahook MY.
MIGS: Advances in Glaucoma Surgery (pp 17-25).

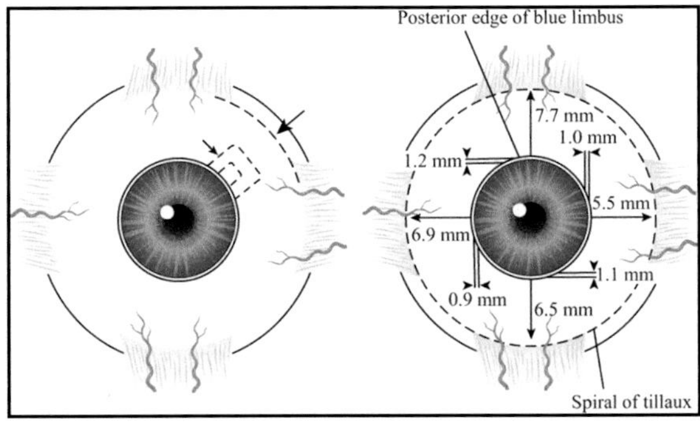

Figure 3-1. The spiral of Tillaux demonstrates the relationship of the extraocular muscles to the limbus, which varies in width as shown here. (Reprinted with permission from Kahook MY. *Essentials of Glaucoma Surgery*. Thorofare, NJ: SLACK Incorporated; 2012.)

rectus inserting approximately 5.5 mm posterior to the limbus, followed by the inferior rectus at 6.5 mm, the lateral rectus at 6.9 mm, and finally the superior rectus at 7.7 mm (Figure 3-1).

The anterior chamber angle recess lies underneath the limbus, an important consideration in scleral-based wound construction. MIGS procedures generally avoid creation of scleral or conjunctival flaps and take advantage of clear corneal incisions to avoid disruption of surrounding tissues.

Conjunctiva

The conjunctiva is a thin, transparent tissue that overlies the sclera and is then reflected along the inner eyelids to form the palpebral conjunctiva. Anteriorly, the conjunctiva terminates at the limbus. Tenon's capsule is a dense collagenous layer found just beneath the conjunctiva that extends anteriorly from the rectus muscle insertions to fuse with limbal episclera a short distance posterior to the limbus. Fibroblasts, macrophages, mast cells, and other white blood cell types are found in tissues proximate to the limbus and influence the wound healing cascade when surgery is performed in this area. While bleb-forming surgeries depend on the integrity and wound healing of the conjunctiva, newer MIGS procedures largely avoid this tissue layer. Patients with scarred conjunctiva due to trauma or prior surgery are often poor candidates for traditional glaucoma filtration surgeries but may still be well-suited for a MIGS approach.

Sclera

Like the cornea, the sclera is composed primarily of type 1 collagen. The random arrangement of scleral collagen fibrils results in the white color of the sclera, as opposed to the transparency of the cornea that results from the organized parallel arrangement of collagen fibrils. Many factors influence scleral thickness, including anatomical location on the eye as well as age, race, and prior medical and ocular disease.[1,2]

Partial thickness scleral dissection is a mainstay of traditional glaucoma surgeries such as trabeculectomy, but is also a key feature of some newer procedures, such as canaloplasty. Although most scleral fibers are relatively disorganized, they become more parallel focally near the location of SC. This is an important landmark used to help locate the canal during surgery involving partial-thickness scleral dissection. The sclera is thinnest, approximately 300 µm, around the insertion of each rectus muscle. It thickens as one moves posteriorly to about 400 to 600 µm at the equator, and continues to thicken posteriorly, becoming thickest, about 1 mm, in the area surrounding the optic nerve and macula.

As one ages, deposition of fat between collagen fibers can cause the sclera to take on a yellowish hue.[1,2] Axial lengthening in pathologic myopia has been associated with posterior scleral thinning.[3,4] Inflammatory conditions that lead to scleritis, such as rheumatoid arthritis, can lead to necrosis of scleral tissue. As a consequence of the relative avascularity of scleral tissue, once inflammation takes root in the sclera, it can persist and become recalcitrant to interventions.[2]

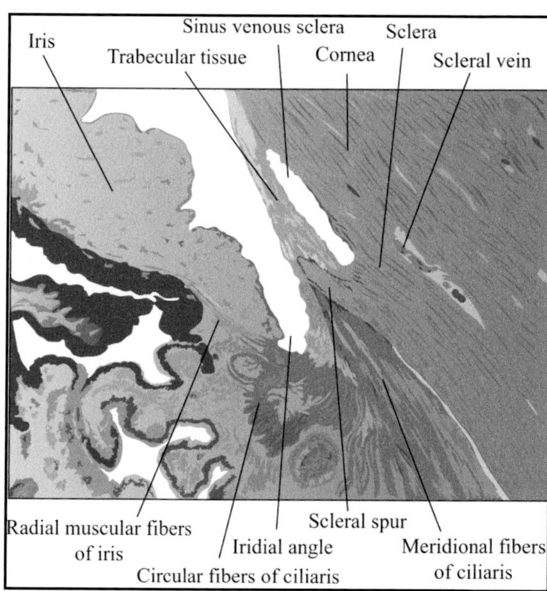

Figure 3-2. Sketch demonstrating the histology of the iris, ciliary body, TM, and SC. (Reprinted with permission from Kahook MY. *Essentials of Glaucoma Surgery.* Thorofare, NJ: SLACK Incorporated; 2012.)

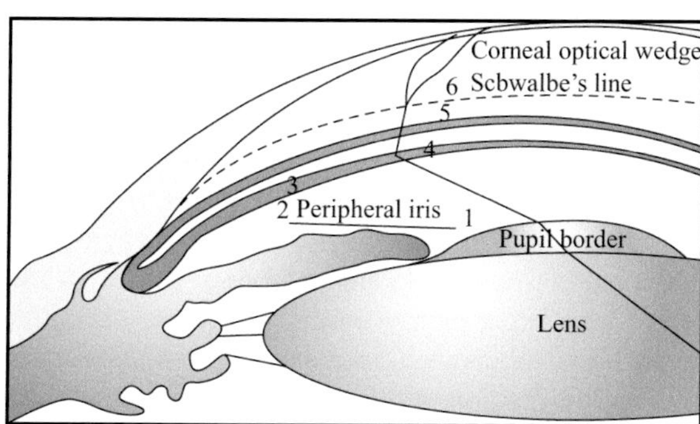

Figure 3-3. Sketch showing the gonioscopic view of the anterior chamber angle and the corneal optical wedge. (Reprinted with permission from Kahook MY. *Essentials of Glaucoma Surgery.* Thorofare, NJ: SLACK Incorporated; 2012.)

Surgical Anatomy of the Anterior Chamber Angle

The anterior chamber angle contains many vital structures that make up the main outflow pathway for aqueous humor.[5] While commonly viewed by physicians during gonioscopy, the angle is seldom viewed in a surgical setting through an operating microscope. Thus, comfort with this view is of utmost importance for surgical success. The angle is bordered posteriorly by the insertion of the peripheral iris root at the anterior extent of the ciliary body (Figure 3-2).

Moving anteriorly, the insertion of the longitudinal ciliary muscle can be seen at the scleral spur. The spur is an important landmark within the angle that is typically identified as the first white line anterior to the iris insertion. The next thin band of tissue anterior to the spur is trabecular meshwork (TM). Using a thin slit lamp beam of light, the angle tissue forms a triangular wedge with the base at the scleral spur and the apex extending to the termination of Descemet's membrane, also known as Schwalbe's line (Figure 3-3).

Histologically, the TM can be broken down into 3 areas that are structurally distinct. The uveal meshwork is adjacent to the anterior portion of the ciliary body and is composed of trabecular beams and lamellae arranged in 1 to 3 layers. The corneoscleral meshwork is deeper and thicker, with 8 to 15 layers of trabecular tissue. The juxtacanalicular tissue is the thinnest of the 3 layers and the least organized, demonstrating loose connective tissue that is not arranged in lamellae or beams.[6] On gonioscopic view, the posterior portion of the TM is typically pigmented to varying degrees while the anterior portion is relatively nonpigmented. Patients with darker skin pigmentation or those with pigment dispersion or pseudoexfoliation may exhibit deeply pigmented TM, while White patients may have very little pigmentation, making visualization difficult. Anteriorly, the angle structures end at Schwalbe's line, the demarcation between TM and corneal endothelium.

SC is distal to the TM. This channel extends circumferentially around the eye at the outer extent of the sulcus created by the scleral spur. The canal lumen is not usually appreciated on gonioscopic view as it is typically collapsed or filled with clear aqueous. At higher episcleral venous pressures relative to IOP, blood can be noted in SC, helping to visualize its location.

Ciliary Processes

Aqueous humor is produced by the ciliary body, specifically the nonpigmented cells of the pars plicata. The pars plicata is composed of the major and minor ciliary processes, folds of tissue that number about 70 to 80 and span the circumference of the ciliary body. They are relatively symmetrical, but can vary in size and shape as well as become longer with age. The ciliary body has a robust vascular supply in the form of the major arterial circle of the iris, which is derived from the long posterior and the anterior ciliary arteries. The arterial circle branches to form a dense capillary bed under the epithelium of the anterior portion of the ciliary processes. The epithelium is composed of 2 epithelial layers, an inner nonpigmented layer and an outer pigmented layer that are apposed at their apical surfaces. The nonpigmented ciliary epithelium is the tissue layer responsible for aqueous humor production and is continuous with the neurosensory retina posteriorly and the posterior pigmented epithelium of the iris anteriorly.[7]

Aqueous humor produced in the posterior chamber passes between the lens and iris and through the pupil to reach the anterior chamber angle. It flows through the TM, starting with the uveal meshwork. It continues through the corneoscleral meshwork, and then passes through the juxtacanalicular meshwork and inner wall of SC. This latter subdivision is traditionally thought of as the primary site of resistance to aqueous outflow.[5] Aqueous humor can also exit the eye via the uveoscleral pathway, coursing through the anterior portion of the ciliary muscle to reach the suprachoroidal space (Figure 3-4).

The outer wall of SC is perforated by anterior and posterior aqueous collector channels that direct aqueous outflow to the distal aqueous veins, after which flow continues to episcleral veins, orbital veins, and finally the cavernous sinus.[8,9] Although supported by septa, SC is thought to represent a potential space with segmented flow and has been shown to collapse with increased IOP.[10] This is postulated to increase resistance to aqueous outflow. Surgical treatment of glaucoma can involve bypassing or stenting this outflow pathway.

Preoperative Gonioscopy

Appropriate management of glaucoma requires close examination of each patient's anterior chamber angle to classify the type of glaucoma (open versus narrow/closed) and help guide treatment decisions, both medical and surgical. This diagnostic measure becomes even more relevant in MIGS. The successful outcome of many MIGS procedures hinges on accurate gonioscopic assessment, leading to appropriate surgical choice and planning. For instance, implantation of a trabecular bypass stent is contraindicated in the setting of narrow angles or angle closure glaucoma. Identification of these types of conditions is critical in the preoperative phase. It is also important to note characteristics of angle structures and pigmentation for each patient preoperatively so that they may be more readily identified in the operative setting.

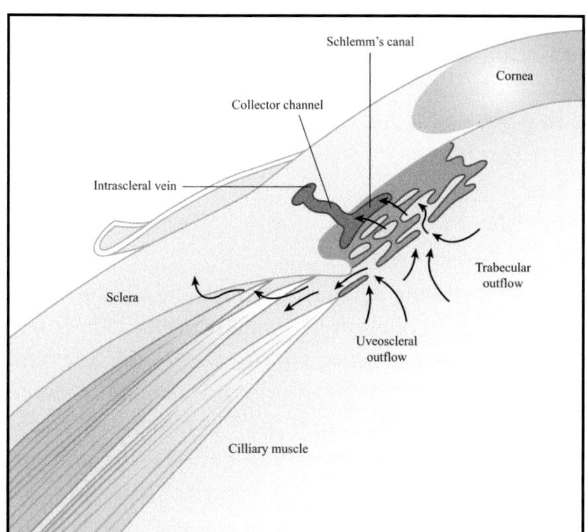

Figure 3-4. Drawing showing the traditional and uveoscleral outflow pathways for aqueous humor. (Reprinted with permission from Kahook MY. *Essentials of Glaucoma Surgery*. Thorofare, NJ: SLACK Incorporated; 2012.)

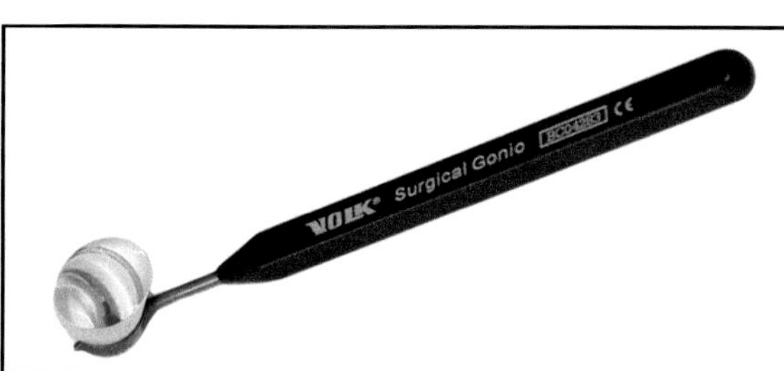

Figure 3-5. Volk Surgical Gonio Lens, Volk Optical, Mentor, OH. (Reprinted with permission from Volk Optical Inc.)

Intraoperative Gonioscopy

Adequate intraoperative visualization of the anterior chamber angle is an essential feature of successful MIGS. Many procedures involve accessing or implanting devices within or near the angle. In the operative setting, this is performed with the aid of direct gonioscopy. As the name implies, direct gonioscopy provides a view of angle structures that is true to life, neither inverted nor reversed. Direct gonioscopic lenses are high-powered convex lenses that overcome total internal reflection to allow light from the angle to exit the eye. It is helpful for surgeons unfamiliar with direct and intraoperative gonioscopy to practice these techniques to ensure proficiency before proceeding with MIGS procedures.

Direct gonioscopy requires appropriate technique and careful positioning of both the patient and the operating microscope. Patients should be screened preoperatively to ensure full neck mobility because the patient's head will often be turned during surgery to achieve the best surgical view of the angle. The microscope will likewise be tilted to allow more direct illumination and visualization of the angle. Traditional direct goniolenses used include the Koeppe, Hoskins-Barkan, or Swan-Jacobs lens. These can be applied to the cornea using an interface of balanced salt solution, hydroxylpropyl methylcellulose (Goniosol, Alcon, Fort Worth, TX), or viscoelastic. Some device manufacturers have developed newer goniolenses with an angled handle to allow the surgeon easy control of their view (Figure 3-5). They are tailored in shape to allow easy access to limbal corneal wounds while maintaining appropriate contact with the eye. These handled devices have laterality, requiring the appropriate choice of lens depending on which eye is being operated upon and the handedness of the surgeon. Use of higher magnification at the operating microscope is typically required to achieve adequate visualization of angle structures. This level of magnification can make entering and exiting a surgical wound difficult and may require multiple adjustments during the procedure. Appropriate viscoelastic use within the anterior chamber can serve to deepen the angle and improve visualization during direct gonioscopy. Excessive use of viscoelastic, however, can collapse SC and make it difficult to access. Lowering the IOP intraoperatively can allow blood to reflux into SC, aiding identification.

Anatomy of MIGS

MIGS procedures attempt to lower IOP by either reducing aqueous production or, more commonly, allowing for increased aqueous outflow. Surgical reduction of aqueous production is targeted at the ciliary processes. MIGS procedures that increase aqueous outflow can exploit several physiologic outflow pathways. Some procedures accomplish this by improving aqueous access to SC, either by removing resistance at the level of the TM or bypassing the TM altogether. Other procedures seek to enhance uveoscleral outflow by creating a connection between the anterior chamber and the suprachoroidal space. In contrast, traditional filtering surgeries, such as trabeculectomy and glaucoma drainage devices, create a novel, nonphysiologic pathway for aqueous outflow from the anterior chamber to the subconjunctival space.

Trabecular Bypass

The main site of resistance to the traditional pathway of aqueous outflow lies at the TM, particularly the juxtacanalicular layer. Therefore, improved outflow to SC can theoretically be accomplished by creating a large, direct passage between the anterior chamber and SC, or by removing TM tissue to improve access to SC. The iStent GTS-100 trabecular bypass device (Glaukos Corp, Laguna, CA) is designed to overcome the resistance of the TM. The iStent is FDA-approved for implantation during cataract surgery for the treatment of mild-to-moderate open-angle glaucoma. It comes preloaded on a single-use insertion device designed to deploy the iStent into SC, creating an artificial fistula between the anterior chamber and SC. The railed end of the device serves to partially stent the normally collapsed SC. While this can effectively bypass resistance at the level of TM, the augmented outflow may be limited to the immediate area around the stent as well as by the number of and patency of downstream collector channels. This may, however, allow for titration of treatment through the use of multiple stents spaced throughout the angle.

The Trabectome (Neomedix, Tustin, CA) uses a proprietary hand piece to strip TM using electrocautery. It is FDA approved to treat glaucoma as a stand-alone procedure or in combination with cataract extraction. During the procedure, the footplate is placed into SC under direct visualization and the device is then advanced along the TM. It is postulated that destruction and/or removal of TM removes a source of resistance to aqueous outflow and allows aqueous to better access SC, thereby lowering IOP. Disadvantages of this technique include intraoperative and postoperative hemorrhage, collateral tissue damage, and downstream scarring of collector channels.[11] Removal of TM also precludes other surgical attempts that are dependent on an intact TM, including trabecular bypass stents and canaloplasty.

Other attempts to remove resistance at the level of the TM include traditional surgeries such as goniotomy. Blades used for goniotomy incise TM to expose SC, but do little in terms of tissue removal. The gonioscraper was developed to accomplish a similar goal of TM removal without the need for electrocautery.[12] Newer devices are being developed that seek to remove the maximum amount of TM tissue with minimal damage to adjacent tissues (Figure 3-6).[13] The dual-blade device is designed to conform to the anatomy of SC, which allows for enhanced removal of TM while minimizing collateral damage.

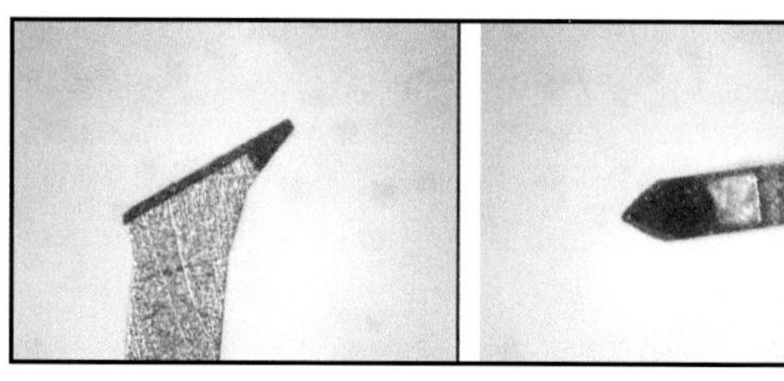

Figure 3-6. The dual-blade device for the treatment of glaucoma.

Suprachoroidal Device Placement

Rather than manipulating the traditional outflow pathway for aqueous, another approach in MIGS is to create a new, artificial fistula between the anterior chamber and the supraciliary and suprachoroidal space as an alternative pathway for aqueous to exit the eye. The CyPass Micro-Stent (Transcend Medical, Menlo Park, CA) is designed to accomplish this task. It can be implanted at the time of cataract surgery or during a dedicated glaucoma procedure. Unlike devices placed into an endothelial-lined space like SC, the CyPass Micro-Stent must be inserted into a potential space between 2 tissue planes within which most surgeons have little experience working. Potential shortcomings of this approach include the propensity to scar, hemorrhage from the well-vascularized ciliary body, hypotony, and failure to accurately place the device in the desired space. By avoiding the TM and traditional outflow pathway, use of this approach is independent of subsequent or prior surgery involving manipulation of the TM.

Schlemm's Canal Expansion/Stenting

Some devices and surgical techniques seek to expand the usually collapsed SC to improve aqueous outflow but do not necessarily create a novel tract between the anterior chamber and SC. Viscocanalostomy and canaloplasty using the iTrack lighted catheter (iScience, Menlo Park, CA) were the first procedures designed with this goal in mind. The former procedure simply involves dilation of the canal with viscoelastic, while the latter seeks to achieve a more lasting dilation with the placement of a prolene stenting suture. However, these procedures require careful partial-thickness scleral dissection that is akin to trabeculectomy. As such, while technically a nonpenetrating glaucoma surgery, they are variably included under the heading of MIGS. Canaloplasty can also be performed using the Stegmann Canal Expander (Ophthalmos, Schaffhausen, Switzerland). Like the Hydrus Microstent (Ivantis Inc, Irvine, CA), it is a fenestrated implant that is inserted into SC to provide structural support and allow for increased aqueous outflow.

The Hydrus Microstent is an example of a newer device engineered to accomplish the same goal but in a fashion more in line with MIGS. The implant is inserted into SC as an artificial scaffold that dilates the canal and allows aqueous to bypass the TM. Implanted at the time of cataract surgery, it dilates approximately 3 clock hours of SC opposite the main corneal incision. This device addresses 2 separate mechanisms of IOP lowering in MIGS: dilation of SC and TM bypass.

Shunting to the Subconjunctival Space

While most new procedures seek to avoid the formation of a traditional bleb, the subconjunctival potential space can still be utilized as an alternative outflow pathway using a MIGS approach. The AqueSys microfistula implant (AqueSys, Inc, Aliso Viejo, CA) is unique in that it utilizes an ab interno subconjunctival approach to IOP lowering. The implant is a thin, flexible tube made of collagen and is designed for subconjunctival implantation through a clear corneal incision either at the time of cataract surgery or as a solo procedure. This novel twist on a traditional surgical outflow pathway allows for outflow to a much larger potential space than other MIGS approaches. Subconjunctival scarring can potentially limit efficacy; in theory, however, this should be less than ab externo approaches to bleb creation that require significant amounts of tissue dissection. Hypotony is also a risk of this full thickness approach.

Endoscopic Cyclophotocoagulation

In contrast to augmenting aqueous outflow, ciliary destruction aims to lower IOP by decreasing aqueous production. Older techniques such as surgical excision, diathermy, and cryotherapy are inherently destructive and lack precise localization of treatment tissue. Thus, these techniques have been largely abandoned or reserved for end-stage glaucoma that is refractory to other treatment modalities in eyes with poor visual potential. Laser cyclophotocoagulation was initially described as a transscleral procedure using a ruby laser, which then evolved to use of the more effective neodymium:yttrium-aluminum-garnet (Nd:YAG) laser.[14-17] Transscleral cyclophotocoagulation is now commonly performed using a diode laser at a wavelength that is more effectively absorbed by the melanin in the ciliary processes.[18] While transscleral laser treatment has the advantage of not being an invasive procedure, without direct visualization of the ciliary processes there is still the potential for collateral damage and an inability to properly gauge the extent of treatment.

Endoscopic cyclophotocoagulation (ECP) was designed to allow for targeted ablation of ciliary processes alone under direct, endoscopic view. The E2 laser and endoscopy system (Endo Optiks, Inc, Little Silver, NJ) combines a diode laser, xenon light source, aiming beam, and video camera into a single intraocular probe. The probe can be inserted through a clear corneal incision or via a pars plana approach to visualize and photocoagulate the ciliary processes (Figure 3-7). Like many MIGS procedures, ECP can utilize the corneal incisions typically used for phacoemulsification, either as a combined or stand-alone procedure.

Wound Healing After MIGS

One of the advantages of many MIGS procedures is the ability to construct wounds, such as clear corneal incisions, that are familiar to ophthalmologists. The more predictable nature of these wounds alleviates some of the difficulties that typically arise when attempting to modulate wound healing after traditional incisional surgeries. The avoidance of conjunctival incisions and decreased dependence on bleb formation may obviate the need for antifibrotics, such as mitomycin-C, to inhibit wound healing.

Nevertheless, the long-term success of most MIGS procedures will still be determined by wound-healing responses. Despite smaller wounds, any surgical manipulation stimulates the immune response and may impact function. Each lumen entrance, exit, or fenestration is a site for possible scar tissue formation that may limit the device's efficacy and cause the surgery to fail. In addition, newly augmented or created outflow pathways will only function to lower IOP as well as downstream resistance allows. Therefore, if scarring takes place at a distal location, any beneficial effect may be diminished or lost. It remains to be seen, however, what effect natural inflammatory and wound healing cascades within the eye will have on these newer procedures and devices. As longer-term data become available, modifications may be made to devices and/or surgical technique to combat these potential pitfalls. It is likely that future MIGS devices will contain anti-inflammatory and/or antiscarring capabilities that could range from surface modifications to coupling various therapeutic agents to the devices for improved efficacy.

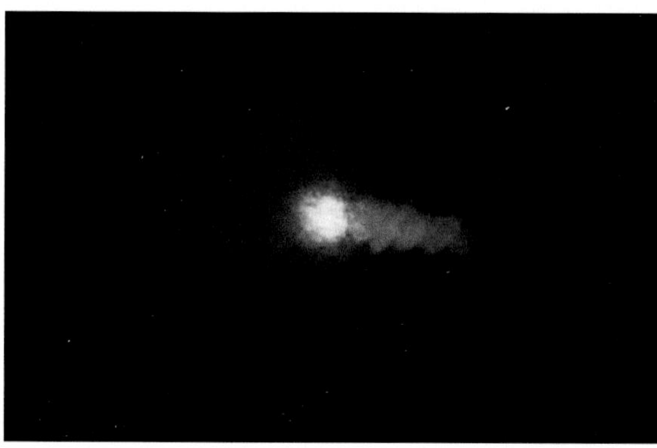

Figure 3-7. Intraoperative photograph of ciliary processes treated with ECP (right side of figure) and untreated (left side of figure). Note the whitening of the treated ciliary processes. (Reprinted with permission from Malik Y. Kahook, MD.)

References

1. Vurgese S, Panda-Jonas S, Jonas JB. Scleral thickness in human eyes. *PLoS One.* 2012;7(1):e29692.
2. Watson PG, Young RD. Scleral structure, organisation and disease. A review. *Exp Eye Res.* 2004;78(3):609-623.
3. Guthoff R, Berger RW, Draeger J. Ultrasonographic measurement of the posterior coats of the eye and their relation to axial length. *Graefes Arch Clin Exp Ophthalmol.* 1987;225(5):374-376.
4. Xu L, Wang Y, Wang S, Wang Y, Jonas JB. High myopia and glaucoma susceptibility the Beijing Eye Study. *Ophthalmology.* 2007;114(2):216-220.
5. Johnson DH, Johnson M. How does nonpenetrating glaucoma surgery work? Aqueous outflow resistance and glaucoma surgery. *J Glaucoma.* 2001;10(1):55-67.
6. Tamm ER. The trabecular meshwork outflow pathways: structural and functional aspects. *Exp Eye Res.* 2009;88(4):648-655.
7. Hogan MJ, Alvarado JA, Weddell JE. *Histology of the human eye; an atlas and textbook.* Philadelphia, PA: Saunders; 1971.
8. Tripathi RC. Ultrastructure of Schlemm's canal in relation to aqueous outflow. *Exp Eye Res.* 1968;7(3):335-341.
9. Krohn J, Bertelsen T. Corrosion casts of the suprachoroidal space and uveoscleral drainage routes in the human eye. *Acta Ophthalmol Scand.* 1997;75(1):32-35.
10. Johnstone MA, Grant WG. Pressure-dependent changes in structures of the aqueous outflow system of human and monkey eyes. *Am J Ophthalmol.* 1973;75(3):365-383.
11. Pantcheva MB, Kahook MY. Ab interno trabeculectomy. *Middle East Afr J Ophthalmol.* 2010;17(4):287-289.
12. Jacobi PC, Dietlein TS, Krieglstein GK. Technique of goniocurettage: a potential treatment for advanced chronic open angle glaucoma. *Br J Ophthalmol.* 1997;81(4):302-307.
13. Seibold LK, Soohoo JR, Ammar DA, Kahook MY. Preclinical investigation of ab interno trabeculectomy using a novel dual-blade device. *Am J Ophthalmol.* 2013;155(3):524-529.e2.
14. Schuman JS, Puliafito CA, Allingham RR, et al. Contact transscleral continuous wave neodymium:YAG laser cyclophotocoagulation. *Ophthalmology.* 1990;97(5):571-580.
15. Beckman H, Kinoshita A, Rota AN, Sugar HS. Transscleral ruby laser irradiation of the ciliary body in the treatment of intractable glaucoma. *Trans Am Acad Ophthalmol Otolaryngol.* 1972;76(2):423-436.
16. Beckman H, Sugar HS. Neodymium laser cyclocoagulation. *Arch Ophthalmol.* 1973;90(1):27-28.
17. Hampton C, Shields MB, Miller KN, Blasini M. Evaluation of a protocol for transscleral neodymium: YAG cyclophotocoagulation in one hundred patients. *Ophthalmology.* 1990;97(7):910-917.
18. Kosoko O, Gaasterland DE, Pollack IP, Enger CL. Long-term outcome of initial ciliary ablation with contact diode laser transscleral cyclophotocoagulation for severe glaucoma. The Diode Laser Ciliary Ablation Study Group. *Ophthalmology.* 1996;103(8):1294-1302.

4

Trabecular Meshwork Bypass Devices

Sabita M. Ittoop, MD; Malik Y. Kahook, MD; and Leonard K. Seibold, MD

One of the goals of MIGS is to induce minimal disruption of the normal anatomy, while optimizing normal physiologic outflow to result in a significant reduction in intraocular pressure (IOP). The principal target is the traditional outflow pathway via the trabecular meshwork. While numerous attempts have been made to augment outflow at this location through laser treatment or tissue incision and removal, this chapter will focus on a device specifically engineered to bypass any obstruction at the level of the trabecular meshwork, the iStent Trabecular Micro-Bypass (Glaukos Corporation, Laguna Hills, CA).[1]

The iStent

The Food and Drug Administration (FDA) approved the iStent in June 2012 for the treatment of mild-to-moderate open-angle glaucoma (OAG). It is a trabecular meshwork bypass device that is to be implemented in conjunction with cataract surgery.[2] Currently, the iStent is the smallest medical device to be implanted in the human body. The device is an L-shaped stent that is made from surgical-grade nonferromagnetic titanium, which is heparin coated to facilitate self-priming. The most recent model (Figure 4-1) is 1 mm in length, with a height of 0.33 mm and weighs 60 µg. The foot plate resides in Schlemm's canal (SC) whereas the snorkel portion resides in the anterior chamber and is 0.25-mm long with a 120-µm bore diameter. The iStent allows a bypass tract through the focal resistance of the juxtacanalicular meshwork and facilitates conventional outflow.[1,2]

The iStent was designed based on the trabecular bypass flow hypothesis. Aqueous humor flows from the anterior chamber through the trabecular meshwork to enter SC and is drained by collector channels into the episcleral veins. For patients with primary open-angle glaucoma (POAG), the juxtacanalicular meshwork is believed to be the primary location for the resistance to outflow. A trabecular bypass tract allows for a pathway of negligible resistance for aqueous humor to pass into SC (Figure 4-2). This causes an increase in the pressure applied directly on the downstream collector channels and subsequently increases the aqueous drainage into the episcleral veins, especially in the quadrant where the bypass is located. This theory has been supported by in vitro studies.[3,4]

Kahook MY.
MIGS: Advances in Glaucoma Surgery (pp 27-35).

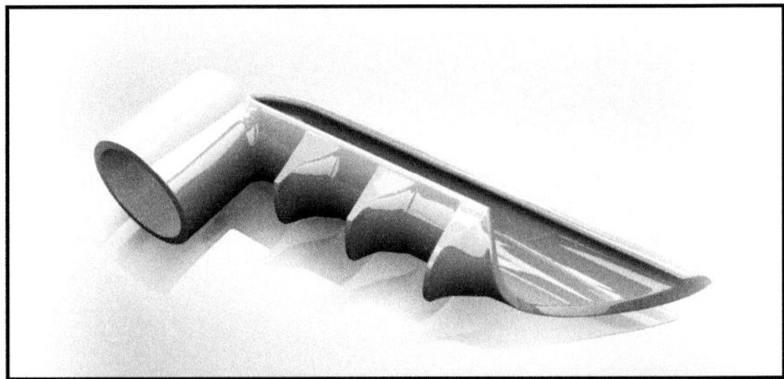

Figure 4-1. iStent Trabecular Micro-Bypass device. (Reprinted with permission from Glaukos Corporation.)

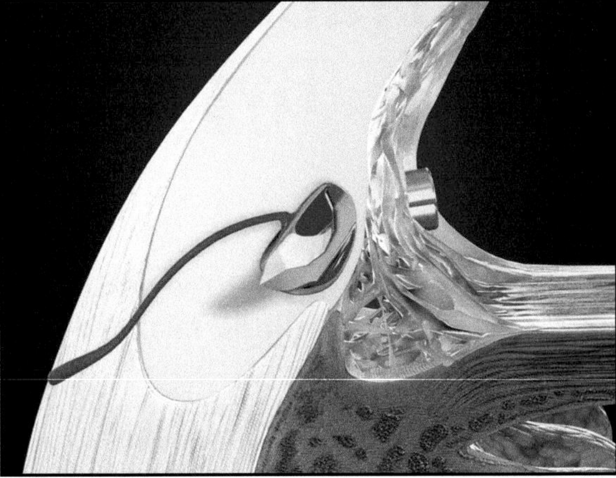

Figure 4-2. Schematic of a well-positioned iStent serving as a trabecular micro-bypass tract for aqueaous humor to pass directly into SC where it can then pass to downstream collector channels. (Reprinted with permission from Glaukos Corporation.)

Patient Selection

The FDA specifically approved the iStent for patients with visually significant cataracts and coexisting mild-to-moderate OAG currently treated with ocular hypotensive medication.

Preliminary studies have shown a benefit in some patients with pigmentary and pseudoexfoliative OAG[5,6] as well as steroid-induced and traumatic glaucoma.[7,8] For these patients, the effectiveness of the device is dependent on the patency of the post-trabecular outflow channels, which includes SC and the collector channels. Considering the high safety profile of the iStent, one can also consider implantation of the device in pseudophakic patients, as a stand-alone surgical intervention; however, this is currently an off-label use of the device in the United States.

As stated in the US directions for use, contraindications include eyes with primary or secondary angle closure glaucoma, and patients with retrobulbar tumor, thyroid eye disease, Sturge-Weber syndrome, or any other type of condition that may cause elevated episcleral venous pressure (EVP),[5,9] since elevation of IOP is dictated by EVP and not necessarily due to outflow resistance at the level of the trabecular meshwork. Warnings include corneal abnormalities that would inhibit a gonioscopic view of the intended implant location.[5,9] Examples include Peter's anomaly, ICE syndrome, posterior polymorphous corneal dystrophy, corneal haze, or corneal opacity. The safety and effectiveness of the iStent has not been established in patients with various conditions including prior glaucoma surgery of any type including argon laser trabeculoplasty and uveitic glaucoma.[9] In these latter cases, inflammatory cells, fibrin, and debris can obstruct the stent.

Surgical Technique

Understanding and identifying the anatomical landmarks of the angle is critical to surgical success. A basic review of gonioscopy as well as in office and intraoperative practice is recommended

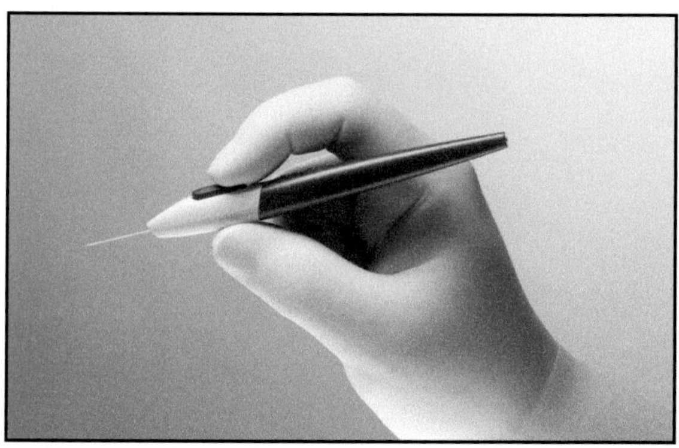

Figure 4-3. iStent preloaded on sterile inserter. (Reprinted with permission from Glaukos Corporation.)

before attempting implantation of the iStent. A review of surgical anatomy relevant to MIGS can be found in Chapter 3.

During the first few cases, a retrobulbar or peribulbar block may be used to minimize patient movement. Also, an intracameral or preoperative miotic is recommended to open the angle.

The trabecular meshwork is identified between the scleral spur and Schwalbe's line and is the site for device insertion. During surgery, as the IOP decreases, there is often a reflux of blood into SC, which assists in visualization. Of note, SC is approximately 270 μm in diameter and will appear flat when viewing through the gonioprism; however, it is actually curved. The most pigmented areas of the trabecular meshwork suggest the location for the greatest outflow and the greatest density of collector channels. These clock hours should be targeted for placement of the device.

To optimize the view, the patient's head and microscope must be tilted at least 35 degrees or greater, where the patient's head is tilted away from the surgeon and the surgical microscope illumination is directed away from the surgeon. The patient is also asked to fixate away from the surgeon. The circulating nurse must be trained to assist as you change positions from the standard cataract setting to the necessary tilt for optimal visualization.

As a stand-alone procedure, a temporal 1.5-mm clear cornea incision is required. During cataract surgery, the standard keratome incision is recommended as this will typically meet or surpass minimum size requirements. Ideally, the incision is made 180 degrees away from the planned insertion site and as close to the limbus as possible. A more anterior incision will obscure visualization with gonioscopy. The anterior chamber is maintained with viscoelastic after the standard steps for a temporal approach phacoemulsification with intraocular lens (IOL) implantation. A dispersive agent is recommended to coat the angle and can be followed by a cohesive viscoelastic to deepen the anterior chamber. Cataract surgery is usually performed at a magnification of 8 to 10x. However, it is recommended that the angle is visualized under higher magnification (10 to 12x) with the operating microscope, gonioprism, and a coupling agent. The gonioprism should be held in the nondominant hand and gentle pressure should be applied to form a contact seal with the coupling agent on the cornea. Any excess downward pressure may create corneal folds that can obscure visualization of the angle. If you are having difficulty identifying the anatomical landmarks, applying gentle pressure to the adjacent peri-limbal sclera can encourage a reflux of blood into SC. Once the anatomical landmarks have been identified, you can remove the gonioprism and turn your attention to the iStent.

There are presently 2 versions of the iStent. Both are preloaded on a sterile inserter (Figure 4-3). The right iStent is designed to be inserted into the right eye and the left iStent for the left eye. This laterality of the device was engineered so the sharp distal end can be inserted inferonasally, to point toward the patient's feet. The inferonasal quadrant appears to be the ideal location since a higher density of collector channels are typically found there. Therefore, implantation at this location should theoretically optimize outflow.

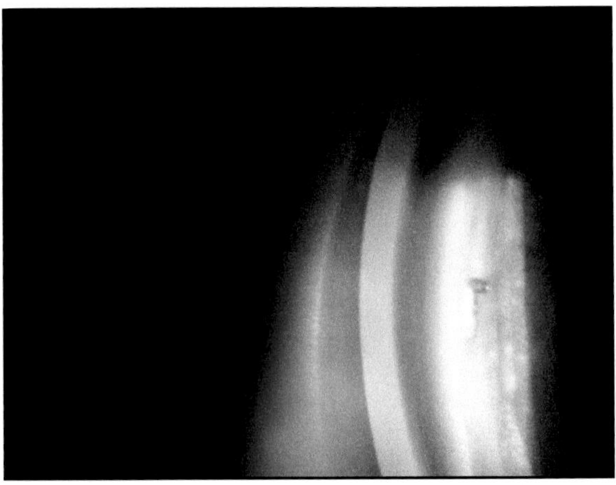

Figure 4-4. Slit lamp photograph of a well-positioned iStent. The inner footplate lies within SC beneath a nearly transparent layer of trabecular meshwork tissue. The lumen of the snorkel extends into the anterior chamber. (Reprinted with permission from Glaukos Corporation.)

Upon entering the eye, care is taken to hold the iStent parallel to the iris plane to prevent iris capture. If the iStent prematurely dislodges from the inserter, it can be easily retrieved and reloaded. When nearing the angle, the gonoprism should be replaced. With the gonioprism in the nondominant hand and the iStent in the other, the iStent inserter is advanced past the pupillary margin to approach the anterior one-third of the trabecular meshwork at a 15-degree angle. The trabecular meshwork consistency is similar to wet tissue paper and thus should be engaged with a gentle rotation as the iStent approaches SC. If significant resistance is felt, inadvertent engagement of the back wall of SC may be occurring. If this occurs, the iStent should be retracted and reimplanted 1 to 2 clock hours away from the original site. The inserter has a push-button release to disengage the device. It is recommended to gently tap the side of the snorkel with the end of the inserter after release to ensure that the device is secured.

Upon examination, the iStent should be parallel to the trabecular meshwork with the inner footplate covered by the trabecular meshwork and the lumen of the snorkel protruding into the anterior chamber. The scleral spur can be a reliable landmark to assess the position of the iStent and ensure that the iStent is seated parallel rather than angled. The retention arches should be slightly opaque as they are covered by the trabecular meshwork (Figure 4-4). If they are visible, a tear through the trabecular meshwork may have occurred or the iStent may be poorly positioned. A small reflux of blood from SC may occur and is suggestive that the iStent is in the correct position. Viscoelastic can be used to displace the blood and visualize the iStent to confirm its position.

The patient's head and microscope are then repositioned to be parallel to the floor. Standard cataract surgery techniques can be resumed, starting with irrigation and aspiration of the viscoelastic. It is important to remove all viscoelastic in the anterior chamber to prevent stent obstruction. Also, a stable postoperative anterior chamber facilitates outflow. All wounds should be checked for leaks and sutures should be placed as necessary. Postoperative topical medications and recommendations are similar to standard postoperative cataract surgery protocols.[2,10]

iStent: Current Outcomes

The iStent was first introduced in Europe in 2004 and most of the initial in vitro and clinical studies regarding the iStent do have limitations. However, the FDA eventually approved the iStent in part because these initial studies consistently demonstrated a significant decrease in IOP with a favorable safety profile for patients with mild-to-moderate OAG. This was later supported by the pivotal randomized clinical trial conducted by the US iStent Study Group, which ultimately led to its FDA approval.[10] Prospective studies with larger study samples are needed to reduce the variability of these results and to demonstrate longer-term trends on IOP as well as optic nerve and visual field changes. Listed next is a summary of the current clinical data.

The first clinical outcomes with the iStent were described by Spiegel et al in 2007.[11] In a subsequent report, the investigators reported their case series of 47 patients with POAG that underwent cataract surgery with one iStent implantation. At 6 months, the baseline IOP of 21.5 ± 3.7 mm Hg was reduced to 15.8 ± 3.0 mm Hg ($p < 0.001$). This was associated with a reduction of topical hypotensive medications from 1.5 ± 0.7 to 0.5 ± 0.8 ($p < 0.001$).[5] Following a similar protocol, the longest prospective case series involves 19 patients with a mean follow-up of 53.7 ± 9.3 months. The study demonstrated an average IOP reduction from 19.4 ± 1.9 mm Hg at baseline to 16.3 ± 4.2 mm Hg ($p = 0.002$), which was determined by the last date of follow-up. This was associated with a reduction of topical hypotensive medications from 1.3 ± 0.5 to 0.8 ± 0.9 ($p = 0.046$).[6]

In the first prospective, randomized, and controlled trial, Fea et al randomized 36 patients to cataract surgery plus one iStent versus cataract surgery alone. The patients were followed for 15 months and topical medications were added systematically if a patient's IOP was repeatedly 2 mm Hg above his or her preset target IOP. At 15 months, the mean IOP in the treatment arm was 14.8 ± 1.2 mm Hg, which was significantly lower than the control group, with a mean of 15.7 ± 1.1 mm Hg ($p = 0.031$). Also, the mean number of ocular medications was 0.4 ± 0.7 in the treatment group as compared to 1.3 ± 1.0 in the control group ($p = 0.007$). In this study protocol, there was a 1-month washout period at postoperative month 15 where all patients were taken off topical medications. At month 16, the mean IOP in the combined group was 16.6 ± 3.1 mm Hg as compared to 19.2 ± 3.5 mm Hg in the control group ($p = 0.042$). No adverse events specifically involving the iStent were reported.[12]

The pivotal US Investigational Device Exemption (IDE) clinical trial was designed as a prospective, randomized, and controlled study conducted at 29 US investigational sites with a sample size of 240 eyes. Enrolled patients were classified as having mild-to-moderate OAG as defined by visual field or optic nerve changes and a medicated IOP < 24 mm Hg on 1 to 3 topical hypotensive medications or an unmedicated IOP ranging from 22 to 36 mm Hg, after a washout period. These patients were randomized to cataract surgery with IOL plus one iStent versus cataract surgery alone. At 12 months, the proportion of subjects with a primary outcome of an IOP ≤ 21 mm Hg without ocular hypotensive medications was significantly greater in the treatment group (72% versus 50%, $p < 0.001$)[10] and remained statistically different at 24 months (61% versus 50%, $p = 0.036$).[13]

The 12-month results also demonstrated that the proportion of patients achieving a secondary outcome of IOP reduction ≥ 20% without ocular hypotensive medications was also significantly higher in the treatment group (66% versus 48%, $p = 0.003$). The proportion of eyes meeting both the primary and secondary outcomes was greater in the treatment group at every follow-up visit. In addition, the Kaplan–Meier analysis illustrates a significant delay in initiating postoperative topical hypotensive medications in the treatment versus control group ($p < 0.001$). At 1 year, only 15% of patients in the iStent group required topical hypotensive medications versus 35% of patients who underwent cataract surgery alone; this difference was significant ($p = 0.001$).[10]

The preliminary 2-year data illustrate that the IOP in the iStent group remained stable from 12 to 24 months with a slight increase in topical therapy (0.3 medications on average), whereas the cataract surgery alone group demonstrated an average increase of 1 mm Hg on more topical medications (0.5 on average).[13]

iStent: Safety Profile

The iStent is astigmatically neutral and was designed to be combined with cataract surgery. Samuelson et al demonstrated that 94% of patients who underwent cataract surgery combined with one iStent achieved a best corrected visual acuity (BCVA) of 20/40 or better at 12 months. This same vision outcome was achieved in 90% of patients who underwent cataract surgery alone. Furthermore, most patients achieved a BCVA of 20/32 or better (85% in the iStent group compared to 79% in the control group). Also, the overall rate of postoperative complications was similar between groups.[10] The overall favorable safety profile was also reported through 2 years of post-operative follow-up.[13]

Conventional outflow is in part regulated by episcleral venous pressure, which ranges from 8 to 12 mm Hg. Therefore, the risk of hypotony is theoretically greatly reduced with the implantation of the iStent as a bypass of the trabecular meshwork. The remaining intact trabecular meshwork ensures a safety net that is bolstered by episcleral venous pressure.[2] As expected, other than one case of transient hypotony at 4 hours after surgery that had resolved by the 1-day exam, no cases of hypotony were reported in the pivotal IDE trial of the iStent.[10]

Regarding complications related to the device, Samuelson et al demonstrated a 4% rate of stent obstruction and a 3% rate of stent malposition.[10] Higher rates have been reported in other studies. Arriola-Villalobos reported a malposition rate of 21% and stent obstruction by peripheral anterior synechiae (PAS) at 10.5%.[6] Belovay et al demonstrated that the most common complication was early postoperative blockage of the stent lumen (n = 8 eyes, 6.1%), which was successfully treated with a neodymium:YAG or argon laser.[14] Fernández-Barrientos et al demonstrated an iStent malposition rate of 18% (N = 33) as their primary complication.[15]

There is a learning curve to implanting the iStent device, and complication rates, in regard to iStent malposition, can be reduced with experience. Also, techniques can be explored to treat stent obstruction due to hyphema or PAS, such as laser, topical therapy, intracameral tissue plasminogen activator, or iridoplasty.

In summary, the clinical studies of the iStent have consistently demonstrated that there is a greater IOP reduction when the iStent is combined with cataract surgery compared to cataract surgery alone. The outcome measures have highlighted that the 12- to 24-month postoperative mean IOP was less than 17 mm Hg on fewer topical medications. Final BCVA was not compromised. The results also supported the high safety profile of the iStent by reporting similar complication rates to cataract surgery alone. There were no reported cases of hypotony at postoperative day 1 or later associated with the iStent and the few complications mentioned were stent obstruction or malposition and reflux bleeding from SC.[16] The surgical procedure for the iStent spares the conjunctiva and preserves the potential for future treatment options. With its modest reduction in IOP and high safety profile, the iStent is an ideal alternative for patients with early-to-moderate OAG who want to reduce the burden of topical polypharmacy treatment regimens and delay the need for filtering surgeries.

iStent: The Impact of Multiple iStents on Intraocular Pressure Reduction

The primary outcome for most of the early clinical trials was whether one iStent combined with cataract surgery produced a significantly greater reduction in IOP when compared to cataract surgery alone. Samuelson et al defined more stringent criteria for their endpoints, with a primary outcome of IOP ≤ 21 mm Hg and secondary outcome of an IOP reduction ≥ 20% without ocular hypotensive medications.[10] Some patients still required the titration of topical hypotensive medications to reach their preset target IOP. This begs the question of whether multiple iStents would allow patients to achieve their target IOP and further reduce or even eliminate the need for postoperative topical medications. This may allow surgeons to titrate the amount of IOP reduction by placing additional stents based on preoperative IOP levels and target IOP.

Belovay et al reported outcomes on patients who underwent a combined cataract surgery with multiple iStents. In this case series, 28 patients received 2 iStents and 25 patients received 3 iStents at the time of cataract surgery. The number of iStents placed was determined by baseline IOP and stage of disease. In both groups, 12-month IOP was significantly lower than preoperative IOP ($p < 0.001$). At 12 months, the group receiving 2 iStents demonstrated a mean decrease of IOP from 17.3 ± 4.0 mm Hg at baseline to 13.8 mm Hg postoperatively, and the group receiving 3 iStents demonstrated a reduction of mean IOP from 18.6 ± 4.0 mm Hg to 14.8 mm Hg. The IOP reduction was similar in the 3-iStent group, with a mean reduction of 3.9 mm Hg versus 3.5 mm Hg in the 2-iStent group ($p = 0.78$). However, at 1 year, the patients that received 3 iStents were on significantly less topical medications than patients with 2 iStents (0.4 versus 1.0, respectively, $p = 0.04$). When the data were pooled for patients receiving 2 or 3 iStents, the overall postoperative mean IOP was 14.3 mm Hg at 1 year with 77% of patients achieving the target IOP of < 15 mm Hg. This target IOP was only achieved by 43% preoperatively on topical therapy alone ($p < 0.001$). In addition, 83% of eyes demonstrated a decrease from 2.7 to 0.7 (74% reduction) in the mean number of topical hypotensive medications used at 1 year ($p < 0.001$).[14]

Also investigating the effect of multiple iStents, Fernández-Barrientos et al randomized 33 patients to receive 2 iStents plus cataract surgery or cataract surgery alone. The trabecular outflow facility was measured by fluorophotometry. Prior to surgery, patients on topical hypotensives underwent a washout period prior to their initial fluorophotometric baseline measure. Postoperatively, topical hypotensive medications were added as needed to achieve their predetermined target IOP. At 12 months, both groups demonstrated an increase in trabecular outflow facility rates (CT). However, the postoperative increase in outflow was significantly greater for the iStent group compared to cataract surgery alone (275% vs. 46%, $p = 0.002$). The patients who received 2 iStents demonstrated an increase of CT from a baseline of 0.12 ± 0.03 to 0.45 ± 0.27 μL/min/mm Hg postoperatively, while patients receiving cataract surgery alone increased mean CT from 0.13 ± 0.06 to 0.19 ± 0.05 μL/min/mm Hg. This correlated to a mean IOP reduction from baseline of 6.6 ± 3.0 mm Hg for the iStent group compared to 3.9 ± 2.7 mm Hg for cataract surgery alone ($p = 0.002$).[15]

Although these studies demonstrate that multiple iStents trend postoperative IOP closer to their target goal without topical hypotensive medication, there is a need for more formal randomized clinical trials with clear cut endpoints to quantify the change in reduction between 1 versus 2 or more iStents.

The Future

The iStent Inject is a second-generation stent design developed by Glaukos Corporation that was engineered to facilitate implantation of multiple stents. At present, the iStent Inject is not approved by the FDA but a large-scale US IDE pivotal trial is currently ongoing.[17] The injector is preloaded with 2 stents and has been designed to facilitate multiple stent implantations without having to leave the eye and to improve ease of device placement. Also, the design of the stent has been modified from the original iStent, although its principal function is similar, and allows a bypass tract through the focal resistance of the trabecular meshwork facilitating conventional outflow.[18]

In vitro studies have demonstrated the second-generation iStent's effect on facility of outflow in human anterior chambers that were cultured from donor eyes. The insertion of one iStent Inject increased outflow facility within 6 hours of implantation from 0.16 ± 0.05 μL/min/mm Hg to 0.38 ± 0.23 μL/min/mm Hg ($p < .03$, $n = 7$) with a subsequent pressure reduction from 16.7 ±

5.4 mm Hg to 8.6 ± 4.4 mm Hg, which was sustained for a 24-hour incubation period. The addition of a second iStent further increased outflow facility to 0.78 ± 0.66 µL/min/mm Hg (n = 2).[18]

Glaukos has also developed a third-generation device called iStent Supra, which is made of heparin-coated polyethersulfone and has a titanium sleeve. This device is designed for ab interno implantation into the suprachoroidal space. There are no clinical outcomes published to date from the recently initiated US IDE study.[19]

Conclusion

The iStent Trabecular Micro-Bypass stent is the first implantable MIGS device to achieve FDA approval. There is significant evidence that the device can lower IOP and decrease the dependence on ocular hypotensive medications when used in conjunction with cataract surgery for mild-to-moderate OAG. The device presents many advantages to the patient and treating physician, including relative ease and rapidity of implantation, paucity of new instrumentation required, and excellent safety profile. Although not fully validated, there is also evidence that the IOP-lowering effect may be titrated with multiple devices. Disadvantages of the procedure include device cost and inability to lower IOP to the degree of more invasive procedures. Future iterations of the device may lead to improved outcomes as well. Continued study of the iStent may expand its role in the treatment of glaucoma and provide surgeons a valuable tool for the treatment of mild-to-moderate glaucoma.

References

1. iStent Product Information. Glaukos Corporation Web site. http://www.glaukos.com/istent. Accessed: May 8 2013.
2. Glaukos iStent® Trabecular Micro-Bypass Stent FDA Approval Information. U.S. Food and Drug Administration Web site. http://www.fda.gov/MedicalDevices/ProductsandMedicalProcedures/DeviceApprovalsandClearances/Recently-ApprovedDevices/ucm312053.htm. Accessed May 8, 2013.
3. Zhou J, Smedley GT. A trabecular bypass flow hypothesis. *J Glaucoma.* 2005;14(1):74-83.
4. Zhou J, Smedley GT. Trabecular bypass: effect of schlemm canal and collector channel dilation. *J Glaucoma.* 2006;15(5):446-55.
5. Spiegel D, García-Feijoó J, García-Sánchez J, Lamielle H. Coexistent primary open-angle glaucoma and cataract: preliminary analysis of treatment by cataract surgery and the iStent trabecular micro-bypass stent. *Adv Ther.* 2008;25(5):453-464.
6. Arriola-Villalobos P, Martínez-de-la-Casa JM, Díaz-Valle D, Fernández-Pérez C, García-Sánchez J, García-Feijoó J. Combined iStent trabecular micro-bypass stent implantation and phacoemulsification for coexistent open-angle glaucoma and cataract: a long-term study. *Br J Ophthalmol.* 2012;96(5):645-649.
7. Morales-Fernandez L, Martinez-De-La-Casa JM, Garcia-Feijoo J, Diaz Valle D, Arriola-Villalobos P, Garcia-Sanchez J. Glaukos(®) trabecular stent used to treat steroid-induced glaucoma. *Eur J Ophthalmol.* 2012;22(4):670-673.
8. Buchacra O, Duch S, Milla E, Stirbu O. One-year analysis of the iStent trabecular microbypass in secondary glaucoma. *Clin Ophthalmol.* 2011;5:321-326.
9. iStent® Trabecular Micro-Bypass Stent [package insert]. Laguna Hills, CA: Glaukos Corporation. 2010.
10. Samuelson TW, Katz LJ, Wells JM, Duh YJ, Giamporcaro JE; US iStent Study Group. Randomized evaluation of the trabecular micro-bypass stent with phacoemulsification in patients with glaucoma and cataract. *Ophthalmology.* 2011;118(3):459-467.
11. Spiegel D, Wetzel W, Haffner DS, Hill RA. Initial clinical experience with the trabecular micro-bypass stent in patients with glaucoma. *Adv Ther.* 2007;24:161-170.
12. Fea AM. Phacoemulsification versus phacoemulsification with micro-bypass stent implantation in primary open-angle glaucoma: randomized double-masked clinical trial. *J Cataract Refract Surg.* 2010;36(3):407-412.
13. Craven ER, Katz LJ, Wells JM, Giamporcaro JE; iStent Study Group. Cataract surgery with trabecular micro-bypass stent implantation in patients with mild-to-moderate open-angle glaucoma and cataract: two-year follow-up. *J Cataract Refract Surg.* 2012;38(8):1339-1345.

14. Belovay GW, Naqi A, Chan BJ, Rateb M, Ahmed II. Using multiple trabecular micro-bypass stents in cataract patients to treat open-angle glaucoma. *J Cataract Refract Surg.* 2012;38(11):1911-1917.
15. Fernández-Barrientos Y, García-Feijoó J, Martínez-de-la-Casa JM, Pablo LE, Fernández-Pérez C, García Sánchez J. Fluorophotometric study of the effect of the glaukos trabecular microbypass stent on aqueous humor dynamics. *Invest Ophthalmol Vis Sci.* 2010;51(7):3327-3332.
16. Minckler DS, Hill RA. Use of novel devices for control of intraocular pressure. *Exp Eye Res.* 2009;88(4):792-798.
17. Glaukos Corporation. GTS400 Stent Implantation in Conjunction With Cataract Surgery in Subjects With Open-angle Glaucoma [clinical trial NCT01052558]. http://clinicaltrials.gov/ct2/show/NCT01052558.
18. Bahler CK, Hann CR, Fjield T, Haffner D, Heitzmann H, Fautsch MP. Second-generation trabecular meshwork bypass stent (iStent inject) increases outflow facility in cultured human anterior segments. *Am J Ophthalmol.* 2012;153(6):1206-1213.
19. Glaukos Corporation. Multicenter Investigation of the Glaukos® Suprachoroidal Stent Model G3 In Conjunction With Cataract Surgery [clinical trial NCT01461278]. http://clinicaltrials.gov/ct2/show/NCT01461278. Accessed May 8, 2013.

5

Schlemm's Canal Devices

Thomas W. Samuelson, MD; Andrew Schieber, MSME; Kuldev Singh, MD, MPH; and Carol B. Toris, PhD

With the development of several new small-incision, ab interno devices over the past decade, glaucoma surgery is in the midst of a renaissance. Surgery for glaucomatous disease refractory to medical and laser therapy continues to evolve slowly with trabeculectomy and drainage device implantation remaining the standard procedures for such patients. The shortcomings of these surgeries, primarily due to postoperative complications involving the surgical drainage bleb, are well documented. The new class of MIGS devices enhance conventional outflow pathways, typically via Schlemm's canal (SC)or the suprachoroidal space. For these reasons, MIGS devices are particularly amenable to combination with cataract surgery.[1]

An estimated 10% to 20% of the 3 million patients undergoing cataract surgery in the United States are receiving IOP-lowering medications for glaucoma, most of whom are in early stages of the disease. This constitutes a large group of patients who might be eligible for a combined cataract and glaucoma surgical procedure, presenting an opportunity to favorably change the trajectory of glaucomatous disease.[2] If shown effective, these devices may lead to a revolution in the surgical treatment of early stage glaucoma.

The Hydrus Microstent (Ivantis Inc, Irvine, CA) is a MIGS device designed for implantation into SC via an ab interno approach (Figure 5-1A). Using a hand-held inserter (Figure 5-1B), the Hydrus Microstent can be positioned within the canal through a clear corneal incision as small as 1.5 mm, making the device fully compatible with modern small incision cataract surgery and phacoemulsification. Once in place, the microstent provides a scaffold for SC thereby allowing access to multiple collector channels that drain the aqueous humour from the trabecular meshwork (TM). The Hydrus Microstent is composed of Nitinol (Nitinol Devices & Components, Inc, Fremont, CA), a highly elastic and biocompatible material that is used in cardiovascular implants. Both laboratory and clinical investigations regarding the Hydrus Microstent have been positive to date and there is much excitement and optimism amongst many in the glaucoma community that this device will allow the ophthalmologist to better treat patients with glaucomatous disease.

Kahook MY.
MIGS: Advances in Glaucoma Surgery (pp 37-45).

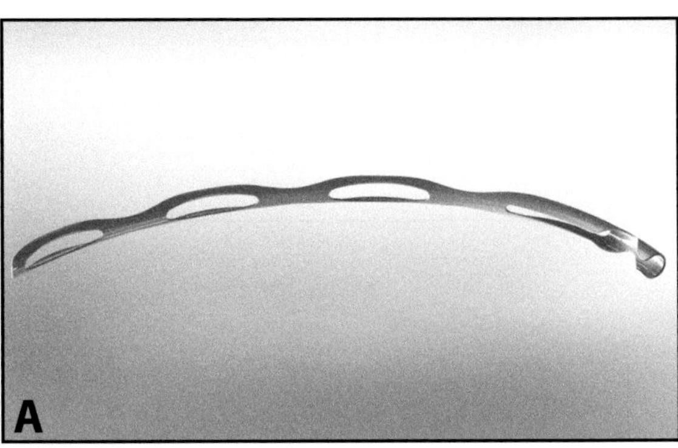

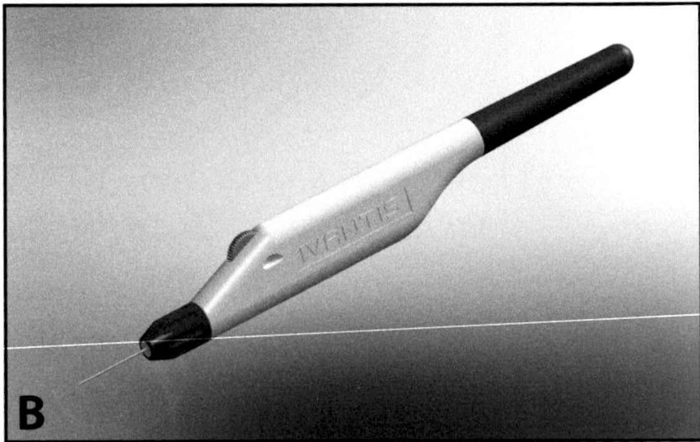

Figure 5-1. (A) The Hydrus Microstent. (B) Hand-held insertion device. (Reprinted with permission from Ivantis, Inc.)

History and Initial Design Concepts

There are several known approaches to improving outflow through the conventional pathway via SC. The goal of each of these approaches is to increase aqueous fluid drainage via the episcleral veins without construction of a bleb for fluid egress, the most common source of postoperative complications related to filtration surgery, such as dysesthesia, ocular infection, and hypotony.

The Hydrus Microstent was conceptualized to increase and sustain conventional outflow by creating an opening in the TM to eliminate the problem of TM resistance and by dilating a significant portion of SC to optimize circumferential flow to multiple collector channels. Design criteria were set to meet these dual purposes. The first consideration for such a device was to find the appropriate material. Both flexibility and stiffness are required to provide the trackability for implanting the microstent into SC. These properties are found in Nitinol, which is an alloy of nearly equal parts of nickel (Ni) and titanium (Ti). Nitinol is a unique metal in that it has shape memory and super-elastic properties, which make it suitable as a support structure in SC. Nitinol has a proven biocompatibility record and has been used extensively in a variety of implantable devices in vascular and orthopedic applications.[3-18] Second, to minimize tissue disruption and allow unobstructed collector channel access, an open frame configuration was designed to minimize tissue contact. A rounded profile also allows atraumatic delivery of the microstent through tortuous, restrictive passages with minimal force. Lastly, the inlet was designed to maintain the TM opening after implantation and minimize the chances of obstruction, thus providing lasting communication between the anterior chamber and SC.

Earlier versions of the Hydrus Microstent had lengths of 9, 12, and 15 mm and also had nearly circular profiles that dilated SC an average of 188 µm along the entire length and 241 µm at the inlet. Laboratory perfusion studies in human anterior segments using the 15-mm prototype showed substantial increase in outflow facility from baseline.[19] Histological examination showed

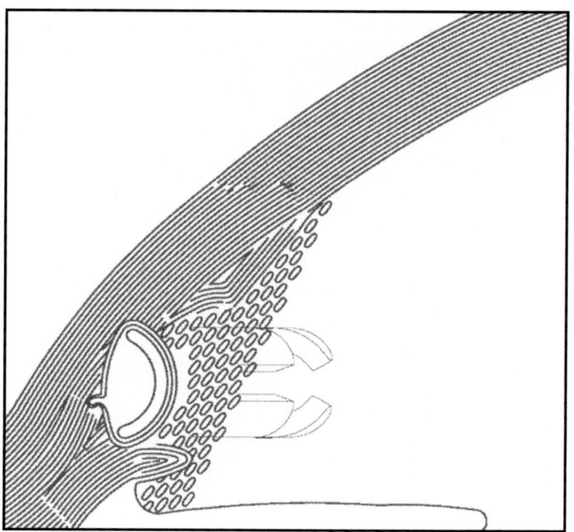

Figure 5-2. Schematic drawing of the Hydrus Microstent within SC. (Reprinted with permission from Gulati V, Fan S, Hays CL, Samuelson TW, Ahmed IK, Toris CB. A novel 8-mm SC scaffold reduces outflow resistance in a human anterior segment perfusion model. *Invest Ophthalmol Vis Sci.* 2013;54(3):1698-1704.)

that the scaffold dilated SC with no visible damage to the TM. However, contact with the back wall of SC was greater than anticipated, potentially obstructing some collector channel ostia. Therefore, a low profile crescent shape having less contact with the back wall of SC was developed (Figure 5-2). Although the 15-mm prototype was deliverable in isolated anterior segments, visualization of the leading edge with gonioscopy during implantation of the microstent was difficult due to device length. Surgical gonioscopy lenses only provide a maximum field of view of approximately 90 degrees, thus only a portion of the 15-mm microstent was visible during delivery.

The Hydrus Microstent subsequently evolved into a crescent-shaped, low profile device that is 8 mm in overall length as shown in Figure 5-1A. The scaffold provides an average of 166 μm of dilation of SC along its length and 241 μm at the inlet. The proximal inlet provides support to the opening in the TM for unobstructed flow into SC and windows facing the TM provide an alternate pathway through the TM. Outflow studies using the 8-mm microstent showed a similar increase in outflow facility to the 15-mm microstent.[20] Scanning electron microscopy of cadaver eyes implanted with the lower profile 8-mm microstent showed nearly undisturbed collector channel ostia. Reducing the size of the microstent did not sacrifice outflow, and the shorter length offered the benefit of a nearly full gonioscopic view during implantation.

Preclinical Testing

Prior to use in humans, preclinical testing was performed on animal and cadaver eyes to evaluate the biocompatibility and functionality of the Hydrus Microstent. As described previously, the Hydrus Microstent is made from a nickel titanium alloy (Nitinol) with unique super-elastic mechanical properties. This material has been used for decades for cardiovascular implants, but the biocompatibility of the microstent needed to be assessed in ocular tissues. Two animal models were evaluated for this purpose.

The microstent was surgically inserted into the SC of 2 healthy cynomolgus monkeys (*Macaca fascicularis*) and a third animal served as a surgical sham control. After surgery, regular periodic slit lamp examination, indirect ophthalmoscopy, and intraocular pressure (IOP) measurements were performed without abnormal findings. At 13 weeks postprocedure, the animals were sacrificed and the eyes were harvested and preserved in a fixative. One eye was examined by light and scanning electron microscopy (SEM). The microstent was found to be located within

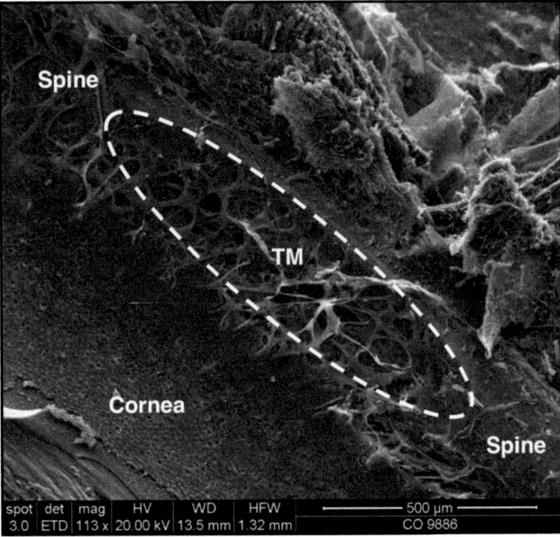

Figure 5-3. Microstent in SC of a nonhuman primate eye. Implantation had been done 13 weeks prior to enucleation and fixation. The dotted line outlines a "window" in the microstent.

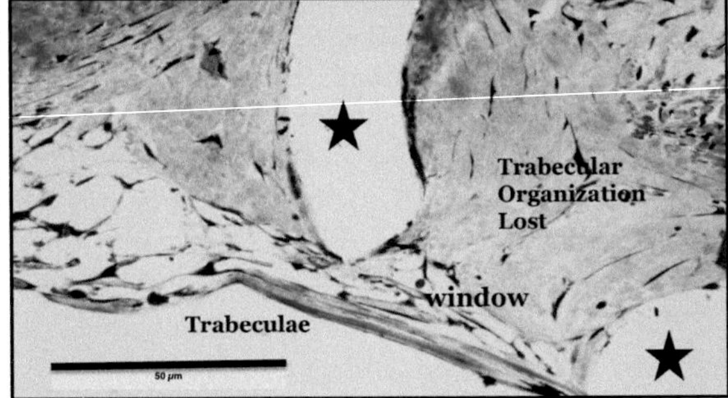

Figure 5-4. Close-up of microstent cross-section in primate eye. No histopathological evidence of metallosis such as depigmentation, apoptosis, or tissue necrosis was present. The host response to the implanted microstent was the presence of a few mononuclear cells with no marked granulomatous response and an absence of giant cells in the adjacent tissue.

SC (Figure 5-3) with its inlet located in the anterior chamber as intended. The microstent had clearly stretched the TM and dilated SC. After removal of the microstent, SC appeared patent. The second implanted eye and a control eye underwent histological sectioning and hematoxylin and eosin staining. An analysis by 2 independent pathologists reported no evidence of an acute or chronic inflammatory response, granulation response or fibrosis in the outflow system, or in adjacent tissues. There was no evidence of tissue degeneration adjacent to the microstent or anywhere within the eyes, and no histopathological evidence of metallosis such as depigmentation, apoptosis, or tissue necrosis. The host response to the microstent was limited to the presence of a few mononuclear cells with no marked granulomatous response and an absence of giant cells in the adjacent tissue.[21] A representative histopathologic section is shown in Figure 5-4.

Additionally, Hydrus Microstents were inserted in the eyes of 8 rabbits through the anterior chamber and positioned to be in contact with the sclera, conjunctiva, and orbital tissue. The fellow eye of each rabbit underwent a sham procedure without microstent placement. Slit lamp examinations were conducted during a 6-month period to observe any ocular changes. After the initial postoperative anterior chamber inflammatory response and bleeding were resolved, no significant findings were noted. The rabbits were sacrificed and histological examination of cross-sections by light microscopy was performed. Minimal mononuclear cell infiltration and minimal fibrotic response at the site of the microstents were observed, even in the highly vascularized and reactive tissues of the conjunctiva and orbit (Figure 5-5).

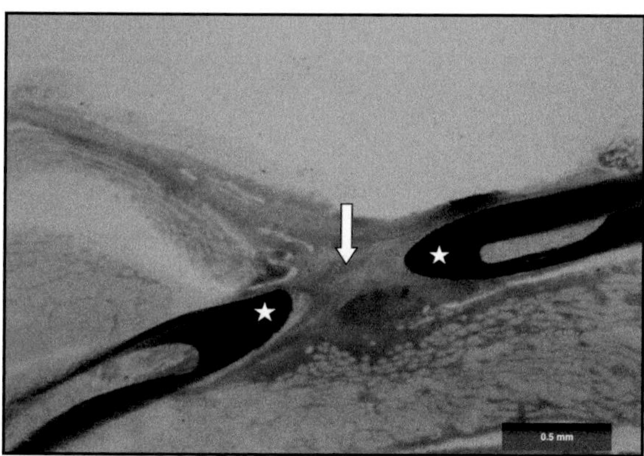

Figure 5-5. Cross-section of Hydrus device in a rabbit sclera showing 2 segments of the microstent (stars) with minimal mononuclear cell infiltration and minimal fibrotic response marked with a white arrow.

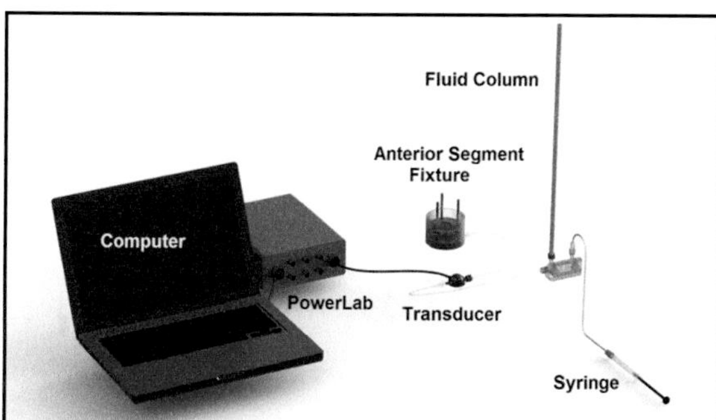

Figure 5-6. Setup for measuring outflow facility in anterior segments. (Reprinted with permission from Ivantis, Inc.)

Outflow Testing

Outflow facility and resistance were assessed in human cadaver anterior segments. In studies of the 8-mm long microstent, anterior segments were isolated and connected to a perfusion system (Figure 5-6). Flow rates were measured at pressures of 10, 20, 30, and 40 mm Hg. The microstent was inserted into SC of experimental eyes, and a sham incision was performed on control eyes. Flow rate measurements were repeated at the 4 pressure levels. From the available pressure levels and rates of flow, outflow facility and outflow resistance were calculated as described previously.[19] An increase in outflow facility from 0.33 ± 0.17 µl/min/mm Hg to 0.52 ± 0.19 µl/min/mm Hg (mean ± SD, n = 24, $p < 0.001$) was found with the 8-mm microstent. Outflow resistance was significantly reduced from 4.38 ± 3.03 mm Hg/µl/min at baseline to 2.34 ± 1.04 mm Hg/µl/min ($p < 0.001$) with the microstent.[20] The potential IOP-lowering effect was higher in eyes with higher outflow resistance (and IOP) compared to eyes with lower outflow resistance (and IOP). Histological examination of cross-sections of regions of the eyes with the microstent showed widely dilated SCs in comparison to the SC regions without the microstent. TM tissue adjacent to the microstent appeared to be compressed but remained intact (Figure 5-7).

To assess outflow patterns, a fixed volume (0.3 mL) of fluorescent tracer microspheres (200 nm, 0.002%), was perfused into the anterior chamber of each eye at 23 mm Hg. Perfusate was collected, and tracer distribution in the TM and episcleral veins was imaged globally. The study showed that less tracer was found in the TM of eyes with the Hydrus Microstent than in the control eyes ($p = 0.0043$). The Hydrus Microstent significantly increased the total amount of tracer flowing into the episcleral veins and perfusate, which drained out of the eye, compared to control eyes (58% versus 35%, $p = 0.0043$).[22]

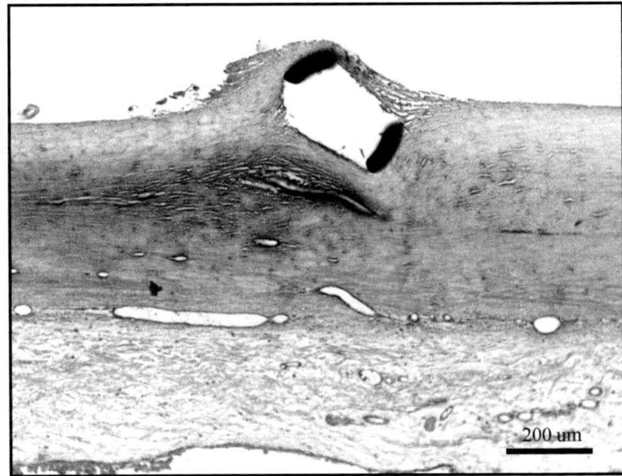

Figure 5-7. Cross-section of the Hydrus Microstent in SC of a human cadaver eye. SC is dilated and the TM is stretched but visibly intact. (Reprinted with permission from Gulati V, Fan S, Hays CL, Samuelson TW, Ahmed IK, Toris CB. A novel 8-mm SC scaffold reduces outflow resistance in a human anterior segment perfusion model. *Invest Ophthalmol Vis Sci.* 2013;54(3):1698-1704.)

Human Cadaver Eyes

The structural effects of the microstent on the anatomy of the outer wall of SC and the collector channel ostia were evaluated by SEM in fresh human cadaver anterior segments. Images were examined for irregular particulate matter, the shape of the collector channel ostia, and the surface anatomy of the SC endothelium. Results showed significant dilation of SC and intact TM. Collector channel ostia along the back wall of SC were neither occluded by cellular debris nor closed by microstent compression. The presence of nuclear bulges in the SC endothelium, a marker of cellular integrity, was observed in most eyes with microstent insertions.[23]

Other Preclinical Testing

The Hydrus Microstent was subjected to the battery of tests required for assessment of permanent device implants. Most important among these tests were those pertaining to structural integrity, corrosion resistance, and magnetic resonance imaging (MRI) compatibility. The surface quality, edge quality, and dimensional tolerances were evaluated using dimensional analysis and SEM examination. Corrosion resistance was demonstrated in accordance with ASTM F2129-08 Standard Test Method for Conducting Cyclic Potential Dynamic Polarization Measurements to Determine the Corrosion Susceptibility of Small Implant Devices. Lastly, MRI compatibility was demonstrated in accordance with FDA Guidance Establishing Safety and Compatibility of Passive Implants in the Magnetic Resonance (MR) Environment and ASTM standards.

Clinical Studies

The Hydrus I study was the first clinical trial to evaluate the safety and effectiveness of the 8-mm Hydrus Microstent and delivery device (Figure 5-8). Conducted at 6 sites in Mexico, Germany, and Austria from 2010 to 2011, the study evaluated the safety and performance of the microstent for lowering IOP under a medical ethics committee-approved protocol in which informed consent was obtained prior to study commencement. Major inclusion criteria were a diagnosis of primary open-angle or pseudoexfoliative glaucoma, an IOP of < 24 mm Hg on 1 to 4 hypotensive medications, and mild-to-moderate visual field defect. Secondary glaucomas other than exfoliative glaucoma and significant ocular pathology other than cataract were excluded. There were 69 patients

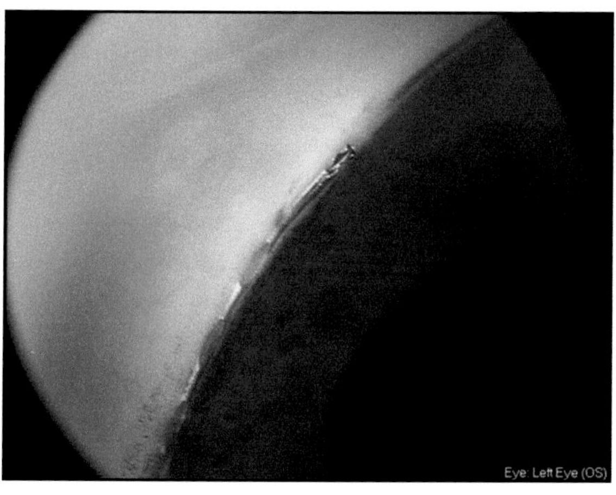

Figure 5-8. Hydrus Microstent in place showing inlet residing in the anterior chamber and the length of the device in SC behind a translucent TM. (Reprinted with permission from Iqbal Ike Ahmed, MD.)

treated within the targeted mild-to-moderate glaucoma population. Mild-to-moderate glaucoma was defined as a mean deviation of no worse than -12 dB based upon perimetric testing. Of this group, 40 patients were treated solely with the Hydrus Microstent device and 29 were treated in combination with cataract surgery. An example of the appearance of the Hydrus Microstent within SC is shown in Figure 5-8.

Preliminary outcomes in this study have been presented at professional society meetings. As reported by Samuelson et al at the 2012 Academy of Ophthalmology meeting,[24] in patients treated with the device as a stand-alone procedure, a mean IOP of 20% was observed, accompanied by a 69% reduction in medication use at month 12. In patients undergoing combined phacoemulsification (phaco) cataract surgery with Hydrus Microstent implantation, 12-month mean IOP was reduced by 33% and medications were reduced by 85% compared to baseline levels.[25] Phacoemulsification has been shown to contribute to IOP lowering, thus the proportion of the IOP drop due to the device compared to phaco alone is unknown. However, further studies comparing the microstent combined with phaco to phaco alone are underway to address this question.

In the Hydrus I study, the majority of complications and adverse events were transient, such as IOP spikes and hyphema, and resolved in the first postoperative month. The most commonly reported long-term adverse event was peripheral anterior synechiae (PAS) observed in approximately 10% of patients at 1 year. In these cases, PAS were small and focal in nature and likely did not affect IOP levels or have clinical significance. No serious or sight-threatening adverse events were observed during the course of the study.

A second study, Hydrus II, is being conducted in 7 sites in Europe. The objective of this study is to demonstrate the ability of the microstent to lower IOP in glaucoma patients undergoing combined microstent implantation and cataract surgery compared to cataract surgery alone. The Hydrus III study is investigating the difference in IOP lowering with implantation of the Hydrus Microstent versus the iStent (Glaukos Corporation, Laguna Hills, CA) when combined with cataract surgery. The primary objective of this study is to compare the efficacy and safety of TM bypass with 3 clock hour SC scaffolding and dilation compared to TM bypass without such substantial scaffolding, when both procedures are combined with cataract surgery.

The Hydrus II and Hydrus III studies incorporate several design features in an effort to control for multiple confounding factors found in glaucoma device studies including (1) medication bias, (2) IOP measurement error, (3) selection bias, and (4) the effect of phacoemulsification on IOP. To control for medication bias, hypotensive medications will be terminated in order to obtain IOP assessment without the effect of these drugs. This process will be repeated postoperatively at the 12- and 24-month follow-up visits and will form the primary basis for assessing the device effect. To control for selection bias and phaco effect, randomization to phaco alone or phaco with adjunctive microstent implantation has been based upon a computer-generated randomization list that is conveyed to the investigator just prior to surgery. IOPs will be assessed by Goldmann applanation tonometry utilizing standardized procedures described in the Ocular Hypertension Treatment Study (OHTS) protocol.[26] Enrollment in the study is complete and follow-up is ongoing.

A pivotal study for purposes of US FDA approval of the Hydrus device (Hydrus IV) is underway in the United States under an approved protocol. Like Hydrus II, this clinical trial is a prospective, randomized, controlled, multicenter study designed to evaluate the IOP-lowering capability of the Hydrus Microstent when combined with cataract surgery compared to cataract surgery alone. This study is also powered to detect adverse safety events as rare as 1% at the 95% confidence level and includes an extensive corneal safety subgroup. After informed consent is obtained, subjects are evaluated for eligibility based on glaucoma status, ocular health, and visual acuity. Refractory patients as defined by a history of prior filtration surgery are excluded from this study. Use of all topical glaucoma medications is discontinued in the study eye for a period of "washout" to establish a qualifying medication-free IOP value. Eligible subjects undergo cataract surgery with phacoemulsification followed by placement of a standard monofocal intraocular lens (IOL). Intraoperatively, after successful completion of the cataract procedure, patients are randomized into treatment or control arms. Clinical follow-up will occur at intervals over 24 months, and complete ophthalmic examinations will be performed to monitor ocular health. At the 12-month and 24-month follow-up visits, patients will be instructed to stop taking all ocular hypotensive medications for a set period of time prior to diurnal IOP assessment. This study incorporates the same design features as the Hydrus II to minimize the likelihood of outcomes bias.

Conclusion

The Hydrus Microstent has many desirable characteristics for an adjunctive procedure with cataract surgery. It can be implanted ab interno with gonioscopic visualization of the angle. Scaffolding of SC increases outflow facility of the trabecular outflow pathway. Low outflow facility is considered to be the primary cause of IOP elevation. Histopathological assessment has been favorable to date with the device being associated with remarkably minimal inflammation in animal models. The Hydrus Microstent has been extensively studied by laboratory scientists with regard to mechanism of action and is being supported by a broad clinical investigation program in North America and Europe, including a large pivotal trial for the purpose of regulatory approval in the United States.

The initial safety and performance profile of the Hydrus Microstent has been established, resulting in regulatory approvals allowing implantation in several regions of the world with others expected to follow to allow broad commercialization. To date, over 600 patients have been treated with the Hydrus Microstent, both under clinical investigations and in open registries in countries where the Hydrus Microstent has been approved. There is much optimism with regard to Hydrus Microstent implantation having a major impact on decreasing the burden of glaucoma both in developing and developed countries as a procedure combined with cataract surgery and perhaps also as a standalone glaucoma procedure.

References

1. Choi D, Surамethakul P, Lindstrom RL, Singh K. Glaucoma surgery with and without cataract surgery: revolution or evolution? *J Cataract Refract Surg.* 2012;38:1121-1122.
2. Chang RT, Shingleton BJ, Singh K. Timely cataract surgery for improved glaucoma management. *J Cataract Refract Surg.* 2012;38:1709-1710.

3. Castleman LS, Motzkin SM, Alicandri FP, et al. Biocompatibility of Nitinol alloy as an implant material. *J Biomed Mater Res.* 1976;10:695–731.
4. Henderson E, Nash DH, Dempster WM. On the experimental testing of fine Nitinol wires for medical devices. *J Mech Behav Biomed.* 2011;4:261–268.
5. Haider W, Munroe N, Pulletikurthi C, et al. A comparative biocompatibility analysis of ternary nitinol alloys. *J Mater Eng Perform.* 2009;18:760–764.
6. Shabalovskaya SA. Surface, corrosion and biocompatibility aspects of Nitinol as an implant material. *Bio-Med Mater Eng.* 2002;12:69–109.
7. Bombac D, Brojan M, Fajfar P, et al. Review of materials in medical applications. *Mater Geoenviron.* 2007;54:471-499.
8. Hannula SP, Söderberg O, Jämsä T, et al. Shape memory alloys for biomedical applications. *Adv Sci and Technol.* 2006;49:109-118.
9. Roosli C, Schmid P, Huber AM. Biocompatibility of Nitinol stapes prosthesis. *Otol Neurotol.* 2011;32:265–270.
10. Achneck HE, Jamiolkowski RM, Jantzen AE, et al. The biocompatibility of titanium cardiovascular devices seeded with autologous blood-derived endothelial progenitor cells: EPC-seeded antithrombotic Ti implants. *Biomaterials.* 2011;32:10–18.
11. Verheye S, De Meyer G, Salu K, et al. Histopathologic evaluation of a novel-design Nitinol stent: the Biflex stent. *Int J Cardiovasc Interv.* 2004;6:13–19.
12. Hill AC, Maroney TP, Virmani R. (2001). Facilitated coronary anastomosis using a Nitinol U-Clip device: bovine model. *J Thorac Cardiovasc Surg.* 2001;121:859–870.
13. Balakrishnan N, Uvelius B, Zaszczurynski P, et al. Biocompatibility of Nitinol and stainless steel in the bladder: an experimental study. *J Urol.* 2005;173:647–650.
14. Kujala S, Pajala A, Kallioinen M, et al. Biocompatibility and strength properties of Nitinol shape memory alloy suture in rabbit tendon. *Biomaterials.* 2004;25:353–358.
15. Wever DJ, Veldhuizen AG, Sanders MM, et al. Cytotoxic, allergic and genotoxic activity of a nickel-titanium alloy. *Biomaterials.* 1997;18:1115–1120.
16. Beeley NRF, Stewart JM, Tano R, et al. Development, implantation, in vivo elution, and retrieval of a biocompatible, sustained release subretinal drug delivery system. *J Biomed Mater Res.* 2006;76:690–698.
17. Olson JL, Montoya RV, Erlanger M. Ocular Biocompatibility of Nitinol Intraocular Clips. *Invest Ophthalmol Vis Sci.* 2011;53:5713-5721.
18. Olson JL, Velez-Montoya R, Erlanger M. Ocular Biocompatibility of Nitinol Intraocular Clips. *Invest Ophthalmol Vis Sci.* 2012;53:354-360.
19. Camras LJ, Yuan F, Fan S, et al. A novel Schlemm's canal scaffold increases outflow facility in a human anterior segment perfusion model. *Invest Ophthalmol Vis Sci.* 2012.
20. Gulati V, Fan S, Hays CL, et al. A novel 8 mm Schlemm's canal scaffold reduces outflow resistance in a human anterior segment perfusion model. *Invest Ophthalmol Vis Sci.* 2013;54(3):1698-704.
21. Grierson I, Kahook M, Johnstone MA, et al. In Vivo Biocompatibility Evaluation of a Novel Nickel-Titanium Schlemm's Canal Scaffold. Poster Presentation. AGS 2012.
22. Gong H, Cha E, Gorantla V, et al. Characterization of Aqueous Humor Outflow Through Novel Glaucoma Devices – A Tracer Study. Poster Presentation. ARVO 2012.
23. Johnstone MA, Saheb H, Toris CB, et al. Effect of SC Scaffolding Device on Collector Channel Ostia in Human Anterior Segments. Paper Presentation. ASCRS 2012.
24. Samuelson T, Tetz M, Pfeiffer N, Ramirez M, Scharioth G, Vass C. One year results of an intracanalicular microstent for IOP reduction in open angle glaucoma. Paper presented at: 117th Annual Meeting of the American Academy of Ophthalmology; November 2012; Chicago, IL.
25. Tetz M, Pfeiffer N, Ramirez M, Scharioth G, Vass C, Samuelson T. 12 Month results from a prospective multicenter study of a nickel titanium Schlemm's canal microstent for IOP reduction after cataract surgery in open angle glaucoma. Paper presented at: 30th Congress of the European Society of Cataract and Refractive Surgery; September 2012; Milan, Italy.
26. Bhorade AM, Gordon MO, Wilson B, Weinreb RN, Kass MA; Ocular Hypertension Treatment Study Group. Variability of intraocular pressure measurements in observation participants in the ocular hypertension treatment study. *Ophthalmology.* 2009;116:717-724.

6

Suprachoroidal Devices

Sarwat Salim, MD, FACS

Traditionally, glaucoma surgeries have used a nonphysiologic route to reduce intraocular pressure (IOP). Both glaucoma filtration surgery and glaucoma drainage devices divert aqueous humor from the anterior chamber to the subconjunctival space and result in bleb formation. Although the efficacy of both procedures has been well established in the literature, unique complications have been noted with each technique.[1-5] Consequently, in an effort to enhance long-term outcomes and minimize complications, recent surgical advances have focused on minimally invasive glaucoma surgery with an emphasis on the physiological outflow pathways, either the conventional outflow system through the trabecular meshwork or nonconventional outflow system through the uveoscleral pathway.

The uveoscleral outflow system is composed of the ciliary body, suprachoroidal space, choroid, and sclera. This drainage pathway was discovered over 40 years ago with radioactive tracer experiments in cynomolgus monkeys and later demonstrated in humans and other species.[6,7] This pathway drives aqueous humor from the anterior chamber to the suprachoroidal space because of a natural pressure gradient between these 2 compartments and a high absorptive capacity of the suprachoroidal space. The aqueous humor leaves the suprachoroidal space either through the scleral blood vessels, the choriocapillaries, or the scleral pores into the episcleral tissue.[8-10] Emi et al[11] investigated the hydrostatic pressure of the suprachoroidal space by cannulation studies in monkeys. They found that the IOP in the suprachoroidal space is always negative when compared with the IOP in the anterior chamber (–1 to –5 mm Hg), facilitating a unidirectional flow. While the trabecular outflow system accounts for the majority of aqueous humor egress from the anterior chamber, the uveoscleral outflow system is of potential therapeutic significance as the aqueous outflow can range anywhere from 5% to 54%.[12,13]

The use of the suprachoroidal space as a medical or surgical therapeutic target is not a novel approach. The most commonly prescribed class of glaucoma medications, the prostaglandin analogues, augments uveoscleral outflow either by relaxing the ciliary body or remodeling the extracellular matrix by activating various matrix metalloproteinases within the ciliary muscle.[14-16] Access to this space via creation of a cyclodialysis cleft (separation of scleral spur from the ciliary body) was historically used as a surgical procedure to lower IOP.[17,18] However, the intervention never became popularized due to adverse events like profound hypotony and its related sequelae or abrupt closure of the cleft with drastic IOP spikes.[19-21] Several other techniques using different

Kahook MY.
MIGS: Advances in Glaucoma Surgery (pp 47-55).

materials and space-retaining substances, including Teflon tube implant, hydroxyethyl methacrylate capillary strip, scleral strip, air, and sodium hyaluronate, have been explored to maintain long-term patency of the uveoscleral pathway and minimize complications with surgically created cyclodiaysis clefts but with limited success.[22-26]

With an increasing interest in minimally invasive glaucoma surgery and the advent of biocompatible, miniature stents or shunts, the suprachoroidal space is being reevaluated as a potential therapeutic area of opportunity. Several suprachoroidal devices have been introduced recently, including the Gold Micro-Shunt (GMS, SOLX Corp, Waltham, MA), CyPass Micro-Stent (Transcend Medical, Menlo Park, CA), and Aquashunt (Opko Health, Inc, Miami, FL). While GMS and Aquashunt are inserted using an ab externo approach, the CyPass Micro-Stent uses an ab interno approach.

Gold Micro-Shunt

The GMS is a 24-karat, nonvalved, flat-plate miniature device that is inserted transsclerally to connect the anterior chamber to the suprachoroidal space. An earlier report of gold retention in an eye without associated cellular or fibrotic response ignited interest in using this inert material for intraocular implantation.[27] The device has been refined over the years to yield 99.95% pure gold in an effort to remove impurities and increase biocompatibility. In addition, design modifications with replacement of internal long channels with posts have stabilized the device and reduced its susceptibility to mechanical damage during insertion. The GMS consists of 2 leaflets fused together in a rectangle shape with a proximal round edge that enters the anterior chamber and fin-like tabs on the distal end that facilitate anchorage in the suprachoroidal space (Figure 6-1A). The device is 5.2-mm long, 3.2-mm wide, and 44-μm thick. The GMS has 19 channels or tubules, of which 9 are open with a lumen width of 24 μm and a height of 50 μm. At the proximal end, 60 smaller holes (100 μm in diameter) and one 300-μm hole are present to allow aqueous humor to flow into the device. The distal end contains a grid of 117 holes (110 μm in diameter) to allow fluid to flow out of the device. In addition, 12 anterior and 10 posterior lateral channels further increase outflow of aqueous humor.

Surgical Technique

After a fornix-based conjunctival flap is created, a 4-mm scleral incision of 85% to 90% depth is made approximately 2 to 3 mm from the limbus. The anterior chamber depth is maintained with either a viscoelastic agent or an anterior chamber maintainer. The crescent blade is used to make a scleral tunnel anteriorly into the cornea and posteriorly into the suprachoroidal space. A sterile inserter is supplied with each implant to facilitate handling and insertion. The proximal end is inserted into the anterior chamber with its concave configuration designed to minimize contact with the iris or corneal endothelium. Only 1 to 1.5 mm of the device should be visible in the anterior chamber (Figure 6-1B). The distal end is tucked into the suprachoroidal space with all posterior drainage openings of the implant covered by the posterior scleral lip. Correct position of the device can be ascertained with intraoperative gonioscopy. The scleral incision is closed with nylon sutures, and the conjunctiva is closed with vicryl sutures.

Clinical Outcomes

In a prospective, noncomparative case series of 38 patients, Melamed et al[28] evaluated the efficacy and safety of the GMS. Most eyes had a diagnosis of either primary or secondary open-angle glaucoma. The mean follow-up was 11.7 months. The surgical success, defined as IOP greater than 5 mm Hg and lower than 22 mm Hg, was achieved in 79% of the cases with or without

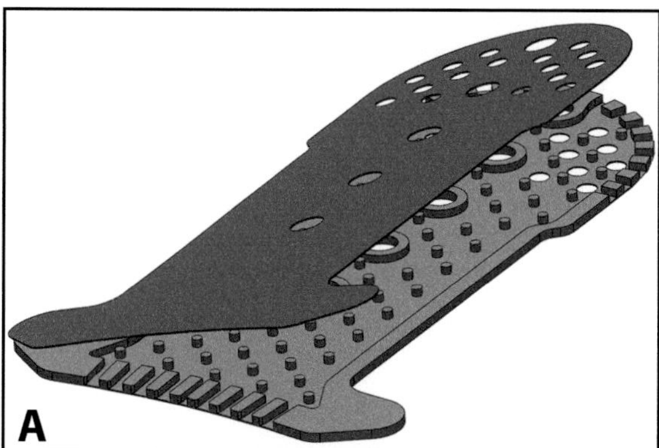

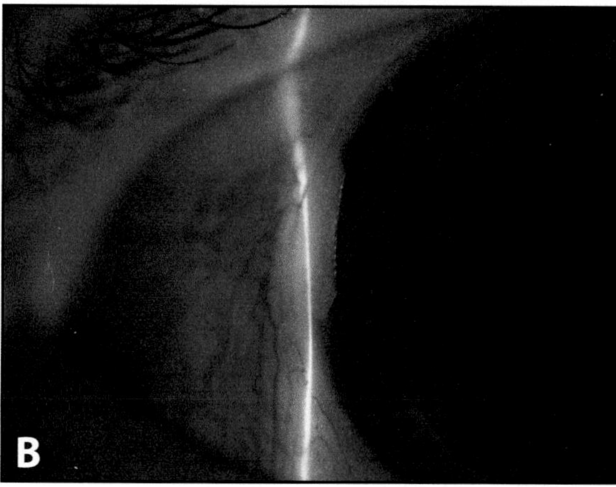

Figure 6-1. (A) Interior view of the GMS showing channels and tubules that facilitate flow of aqueous humor from the anterior chamber to the suprachoroidal space. (B) One to 1.5 mm of exposed proximal end of the GMS in the anterior chamber with temporal placement. (Reprinted with permission from SOLX Corp.)

antiglaucoma medications. Mean IOP was reduced by approximately 9 mm Hg from 27.6 ± 4.7 to 18.2 ± 4.6 mm Hg (P < .001). The most common complication reported was transient hyphema (n = 8). Francis et al[29] categorized this pilot study as level III evidence in support of the procedure in their ophthalmic technology assessment report.

Figus et al[30] reported a prospective, uncontrolled case series of 55 patients with a follow-up of 24 months. Study eyes underwent a mean of 1.9 ± 0.7 glaucoma surgical interventions prior to enrollment and had a mean baseline IOP of 30.8 ± 8.8 mm Hg. At 2 years of follow-up, qualified and complete success rates were reported to be 67% and 6%, respectively. The most commonly encountered complication was self-limited hyphema. The most important factor affecting the efficacy of GMS was development of a thin membrane obstructing the anterior holes in 12 patients (66.7% of failures).

Melamed et al[31] reported 5-year outcomes in a prospective, randomized clinical trial comparing Ahmed glaucoma valve and GMS in patients with refractory glaucoma. The authors used a new design of GMS with posts instead of tubes and a concave anterior design with larger windows. Thirty-two patients participated in the trial; 69% had primary open-angle glaucoma and 31% had exfoliation glaucoma. At 5 years, both groups showed a statistically significant decline in IOP and number of glaucoma medications after surgery. The cumulative probabilities of success were 77.8% for the Ahmed group and 69.6% for the GMS group. The authors concluded that the new design may provide better long-term outcomes.

Mastropasqua et al[32] described in vivo confocal microscopy (IVCM) features in 14 eyes with primary open-angle glaucoma after GMS implantation in the suprachoroidal space. An increase in conjunctival microcyst density and area was seen at the site of successful GMS implantation (defined as a 33% reduction in IOP from baseline with or without medications) compared with unsuccessful GMS implantation, indicating aqueous filtration across the sclera as one of the mechanisms for IOP reduction with this device.

Recently, Agnifili et al[33] reported histological features of failed GMS in an interventional case series of 5 eyes that had undergone shunt placement for refractory glaucoma. Examination of the failed shunts revealed connective tissue accumulation and a thick fibrotic capsule surrounding both the proximal and distal ends, indicating that fibrosis remains a concern even in the suprachoroidal space.

In the United States, the efficacy and safety of GMS is currently being investigated in a large clinical trial.

CyPass Micro-Stent

The CyPass Micro-Stent is a minimally invasive suprachoroidal device that uses an ab interno approach for implantation and avoids manipulation of the conjunctiva and sclera, as seen in ab externo suprachoroidal devices. The device is a 6.35-mm long tube with an outer diameter of about 0.5 mm and a lumen of 300 µm. It is made of biocompatible, nonbiodegradable polyimide material similar to that previously used in intraocular lens haptics. Fenestrations along the device facilitate aqueous humor egress throughout its length.

Surgical Technique

The device can be inserted through a clear corneal incision as a stand-alone procedure or may be combined with cataract extraction. A clear cornea and goniolens are needed to visualize the angle for proper insertion of the shunt, although it may be implanted as a gonio-free technique. Prior to its insertion, anterior chamber depth and angle expansion are maintained with a viscoelastic agent. The device is positioned on a small guidewire that is advanced across the anterior chamber until the scleral spur and iris root are identified (Figure 6-2A). The atraumatic tip of the guidewire facilitates nonincisional dissection until the ciliary body is dissected from the sclera, thereby creating a microcyclodialysis. The curved configuration of the guidewire tracks along the natural curvature of the eye. After correct positioning of the device with the distal end below the scleral spur in the supraciliary and suprachoroidal space and the proximal collar remaining in the anterior chamber, the guidewire is withdrawn (Figure 6-2B). The surgical technique is relatively straightforward with an easy learning curve for less experienced glaucoma surgeons. Imaging modalities, such as anterior segment optical coherence tomography or ultrasound biomicroscopy, can be used to confirm both the position and function of these shunts in the supraciliary space (Figure 6-2C).[34] Areas of hypodensity around the shunt indicate filtration and aqueous outflow. The transcameral approach spares superior conjunctiva that could be used for other surgical procedures in the event of failures.

Clinical Outcomes

A European study involving 81 subjects evaluated the efficacy of the CyPass Micro-Stent when combined with phacoemulsification.[35] At 6-months follow-up, the mean IOP was decreased from 22.9 to 16.2 mm Hg, and the number of glaucoma medications was reduced from 1.9 to 1.3. An IOP reduction of 35% was seen in eyes with a baseline IOP greater than 21 mm Hg. In terms of complications, there were 2 cases of self-limited hyphema and one case of a shallow anterior chamber that resolved by 1 month. No major complications, such as choroidal detachment, choroidal hemorrhage, or retinal detachment, were observed.

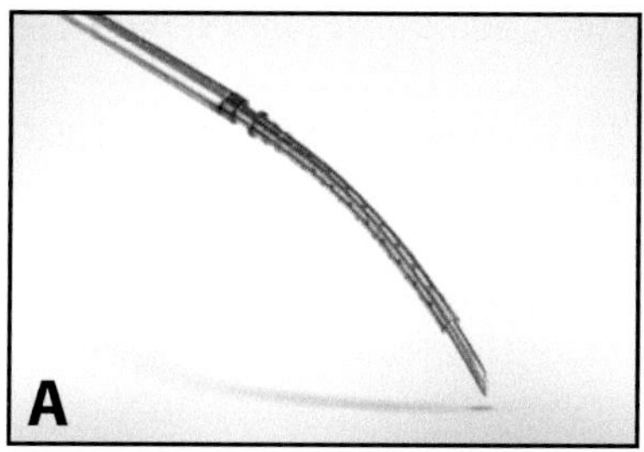

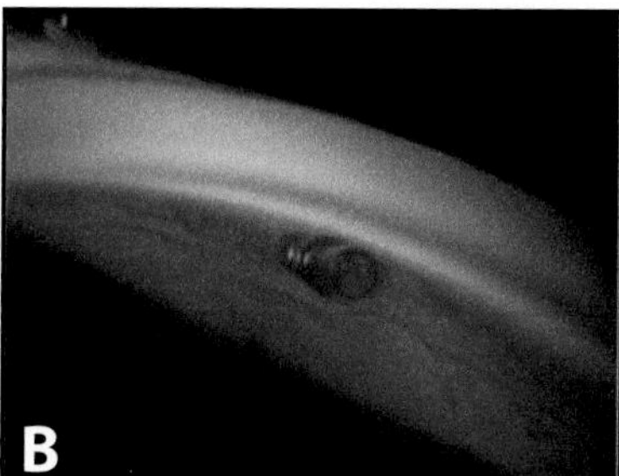

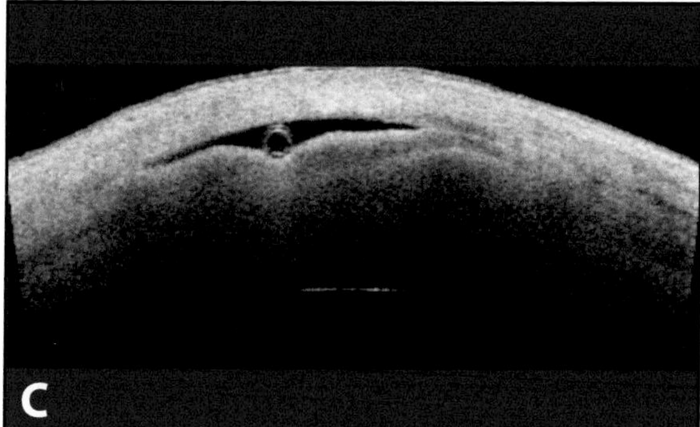

Figure 6-2. (A) The CyPass Micro-Stent positioned on a curved guidewire. (B) Correct position of the CyPass Micro-Stent between the scleral spur and iris root. (C) Anterior segment optical coherence tomography image showing an area of hypodensity around the CyPass stent, indicating filtration. (Reprinted with permission from Transcend Medical, Menlo Park, CA.)

Craven et al[36] reported their experience in 121 eyes that underwent combined phacoemulsification and CyPass Micro-Stent implantation. The most common postoperative complication was reported to be transient hyphema (n = 8). Other rare adverse events included persistent inflammation, branch retinal vein occlusion, and exacerbation of underlying diabetic macular edema.

Recently, the results of the CyCLE Study using the CyPass Micro-Stent were presented at the European Society of Cataract and Refractive Surgeons Annual Meeting.[37-38] The trial enrolled 460 patients: 222 patients underwent CyPass Micro-Stent implantation alone, and 238 received the stent in combination with phacoemulsification. In the CyPass alone group, mean baseline IOP was ≥ 21 mm Hg in 134 patients and ≤ 21 mm Hg in 88 patients. Approximately 50% of the patients had required prior glaucoma interventions, and 27% of the patients had previous glaucoma surgery, either glaucoma filtration surgery or insertion of glaucoma drainage devices. At 12-months follow-up, a 26% reduction in IOP and a 33% reduction in the use of adjunctive glaucoma medications were found compared to baseline values. The most commonly observed adverse events were additional surgery (11%), IOP elevation (8%), and obstruction of the device (4%).

In the combined group, 90 patients had an IOP ≥ 21 mm Hg, and 148 patients had an IOP ≤ 21 mm Hg. Although the number of glaucoma interventions was much lower in this group (11%), a similar percentage of patients had previous glaucoma surgery when compared with the CyPass alone group. At 12-months follow-up, a 33% IOP reduction and nearly 50% reduction in the requirement of glaucoma medications were reported compared to baseline values. The most commonly observed adverse events included device obstruction (5%), additional surgical intervention (3%), and IOP elevation (2%).

Another study evaluated the efficacy and safety of Cypass Micro-Stent for the primary treatment of medication-naïve patients with open-angle glaucoma.[39] The stent was placed in 22 patients through a 1.2-mm clear cornea incision into the supraciliary space under direct gonioscopic visualization. After surgery, the mean IOP decreased 42% and 39% at 3 and 6 months, respectively, from a mean baseline IOP of 26.5 mm Hg. Only one-third of the patients required a single topical glaucoma medication for additional IOP control. No serious intraoperative or postoperative complications were reported.

The CyPass Micro-Stent is currently being investigated in the United States in a large FDA trial, the COMPASS Trial. The results of this trial are widely anticipated to determine additional safety and efficacy of this minimally invasive ab interno stent and its potential role in targeting the uveoscleral outflow pathway. Further preclinical studies as well as postimplantation studies will hopefully shed light on the rate of encapsulation of ab interno suprachoroidal devices. Encapsulation is likely to occur in some patients and innovating successful strategies to decrease the rate and degree of encapsulation might represent a major determinant of success after this intervention.

Aquashunt

The Aquashunt is an ab externo suprachoroidal device that is currently under investigation. It is made of polypropylene material and is 10-mm long, 4-mm wide, and 0.75-mm thick. This device has a large-bore lumen with a 250-μm opening (Figure 6-3A).

Surgical Technique

The surgical technique for the Aquashunt requires insertion through a full-thickness scleral incision to the level of the suprachoroidal space. The device comes with an insertion tool that facilitates its placement anteriorly while keeping the adjacent tissue from blocking its lumen (Figure 6-3B). The shunt is advanced through the suprachoroidal space toward the anterior chamber, shearing the attachments between the ciliary body and the scleral spur and creating a direct conduit between the 2 compartments. After the proximal end is properly positioned in the anterior chamber, the insertion tool is withdrawn. The distal end of the device is tucked beneath the posterior lip of the scleral incision, and the device is secured to the sclera. Both scleral and conjunctival incisions are then closed.

Clinical Outcomes

A pilot study conducted in Central America reported an IOP reduction of 30% to 40% in 13 of 15 cases at 12-months follow-up. Adjunctive medications were required in 6 cases, removal of the device in one case, and further surgery in one case. Fibrosis in the suprachoroidal space was mainly responsible for late surgical failures. Alternative materials for biocompatibility and coating of devices with antifibrotic agents are currently being investigated. As with all suprachoroidal implants, encapsulation is likely to occur in a portion of patients and generating strategies to decrease this process should allow for improved success after this intervention. It is unclear how encapsulation might differ between ab externo and ab interno implanted devices.

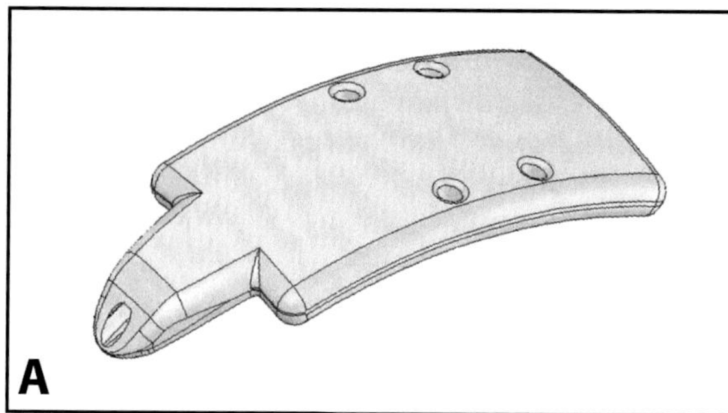

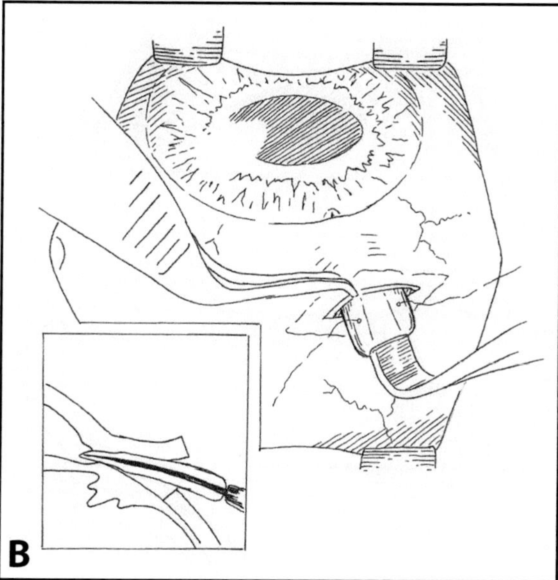

Figure 6-3. (A) Aquashunt device. (B) Schematic drawing of advancing the Aquashunt with the insertion tool. (Reprinted with permission from M. Bruce Shields, MD.)

iStent Supra

iStent Supra (Glaukos Corporation, Laguna Hills, CA) is a new ab interno suprachoroidal device. This 4-mm device has a lumen of 0.165 mm. It is made of polyethersulfone with a titanium sleeve. The device comes with a disposable injector and is inserted posterior to the scleral spur under direct gonioscopic visualization. At present, the device's efficacy and safety are being investigated in clinical trials.

Conclusion

Suprachoroidal devices allow more controlled outflow of aqueous humor from the anterior chamber to the suprachoroidal space. By targeting the physiological uveoscleral pathway, these devices avoid blebs and their related complications. Because glaucoma is a chronic disease that often requires multiple surgical interventions over time, the added advantage of ab interno suprachoroidal devices in sparing superior conjunctiva is of great significance when subsequent filtering surgeries are needed.

While the preliminary studies with these newer devices appear promising in reducing IOP and the requirement for adjunctive medications, additional studies with long-term follow-up are warranted to establish their applicability, efficacy, and safety in various stages of glaucoma. In addition, encapsulation of devices in the suprachoroidal space could represent a significant hurdle for their overall success and requires further investigation of potential causes. Prospective, randomized trials are also needed to compare their efficacy with conventional surgeries, such as trabeculectomy and glaucoma drainage devices, and to determine their efficacy and safety with one another.

References

1. Greenfield DS, Suner IJ, Miller MP, et al. Endophthalmitis after filtering surgery with mitomycin. *Arch Ophthalmol.* 1996;114:943-949.
2. Parrish RK II, Schiffman JC, Feurer WJ, et al. Fluorouracil Filtering Surgery Study Group. Prognosis and risk factors for early postoperative wound leaks after trabeculectomy with and without 5-fluorouracil. *Am J Ophthalmol.* 2001;132:633-640.
3. Sherwood MB, Smith MF, Driebe WT Jr, et al. Drainage tube implants in the treatment of glaucoma following penetrating keratoplasty. *Ophthalmic Surg.* 1993;24(3):185-189.
4. Tessler Z, Jluchoded S, Rosenthal G. Nd:YAG laser for Ahmed tube shunt occlusion by the posterior capsule. *Ophthalmic Surg Lasers.* 1997;28:69-70.
5. Tarbak AAA, Shahwan SA, Jadaan IA, et al. Endophthalmitis associated with the Ahmed glaucoma valve implant. *Br J Ophthalmol.* 2005;89:454-458.
6. Bill A. The aqueous humor drainage mechanism in the cynomolgus monkey (Macaca irus) with evidence for unconventional routes. *Invest Ophthalmol.* 1965;4(5):911-919.
7. Bill A, Hellsing K. Production and drainage of aqueous humor in the cynomolgus monkey (Macaca irus). *Invest Ophthalmol.* 1965;4(5):920-926.
8. Teng CC, Chi HH, Katzin HM. Histology and mechanism of filtering operations. *Am J Ophthalmol.* 1959;47:16-33.
9. Pederson JE, Gaasterland DE, MacLellan HM. Uveoscleral aqueous outflow in the rhesus monkey: importance of uveal reabsorption. *Invest Ophthalmol Vis Sci.* 1977;16(11):1008-1017.
10. Krohn J, Bertelsen T. Light microscopy of uveoscleral drainage routes after gelatine injections into the suprachoroidal space. *Acta Ophthalmol Scand.* 76(5):521-527.
11. Emi K, Pederson JE, Toris CB. Hydrostatic pressure of the suprachoroidal space. *Invest Ophthalmol Vis Sci.* 1989;30:233-238.
12. Bill A, Phillips CI. Uveoscleral drainage of aqueous humor dynamics in the aging human eyes. *Exp Eye Res.* 1971;12:275-281.
13. Toris CB, Yablonski ME, Wang YL, et al. Aqueous humor dynamics in the aging human eye. *Am J Ophthalmol.* 1999;127:407-412.
14. Crawford KS, Kaufman PL. Dose-related effects of prostaglandin F2 alpha isopropylester on intraocular pressure, refraction, and pupil diameter in monkeys. *Invest Ophthalmol Vis Sci.* 1991;32(3):510-519.
15. Weinreb RN, Toris CB, Gabelt BT, et al. Effects of prostaglandins on the aqueous humor outflow pathways. *Surv Ophthalmol.* 2002;47 (Suppl 1):S53-64.
16. Nilsson SF, Sperber GO, Bill A. The effect of prostaglandin F2 alpha-1-isopropylester (PGF2 alpha-IE) on uveoscleral outflow. *Prog Clin Biol Res.* 1989;312:429-436.
17. Fuchs E. Ablosung der Aderhaut nach Staaroperation. *Graefes Arch Clin Exp Ophthalmol.* 1900;51:199-224.
18. Heine L. Die Cyklodialyse, eine neue Glaucomoperation. *Deutsche Med Wehnschr.* 1905;31:824-826.
19. Galin MA, Baras I. Combined cyclodialysis cataract extraction: a review. *Ann Ophthalmol.* 1975;7(2):271-275.
20. Shields MB, Simmons RJ. Combined cyclodialysis and cataract extraction. *Ophthalmic Surg.* 1976;7(2):62-73.
21. Seguro K, Toris CB, Pedrson JE. Uveoscleral outflow following cyclodialysis in the monkey eye using a flurorescent tracer. *Invest Ophthalmol Vis Sci.* 1985;26:810-813.
22. Portney GL. Silicone elastomer implantation cyclodialysis: a negative report. *Arch Ophthalmol.* 1973;89:10-12.
23. Miller RD, Nisbet RM. Cyclodialysis with air injection in black patients. *Ophthalmic Surg.* 1981;12:92-94.
24. Alpar JJ. Sodium hyaluronate (Healon) in cyclodialysis. *CLAO J.* 1985;11:201-204.
25. Klemm M, Balazs A, Draeger J, et al. Experimental use of space-retaining substances with extended duration: functional and morphological results. *Graefes Arch Clin Exp Ophthalmol.* 1995;233(9):592-597.
26. Jordan JF, Deitlein TS, Dinslage S, et al. Cyclodialysis ab interno as a surgical approach to intractable glaucoma. *Graefes Arch Clin Exp Ophthalmol.* 2007;245:1071-1076.
27. Sen SC, Ghosh A. Gold as an intraocular foreign body. *Br J Ophthalmol.* 1983;67(6):398-399.
28. Melamed S, Simon GJB, Goldenfeld M, et al. Efficacy and safety of gold microshunt implantation to the supraciliary space in patients with glaucoma. *Arch Ophthalmol.* 2009;127(3):264-269.

29. Francis BA, Singh K, Shan LC, et al. Novel glaucoma procedures--a report by the American Academy of Ophthalmology. *Ophthlamology.* 2011;118:1466-1480.
30. Figus M, Lazzeri S, Fogagnolo P, et al. Supraciliary shunt in refractory glaucoma. *Br J Ophthalmol.* 2011;1-5.
31. Melamed S, Sagiv O, Simon B, et al. Ahmed glaucoma valve versus gold micro shunt implants--five year results of a prospective randomized clinical trial. 6th International Congress on Glaucoma Surgery, Glasgow, Scotland, 2012.
32. Mastropasqua L, Agnifili L, Ciancaglini M, et al. In vivo analysis of conjunctiva in gold micro shunt implantation for glaucoma. *Br J Ophthalmol.* 2010;94(12):1592-1596.
33. Agnifili L, Costagliola C, Figus M, et al. Histololgical findings of failed gold micro shunts in primary open-angle glaucoma. *Graefes Arch Clin Exp Ophthalmol.* 2012;250:143-149.
34. Ahmed IK, Rau MB, Grabner G, et al. Use of anterior segment OCT for deep angle visualization after microstent implantation. Presented at: European Society of Cataract and Refractive Surgeons; 2012; Milan, Italy.
35. Ianchulev T, Ahmed IK, Hoeh HR, et al. Minimally invasive ab interno suprachoroidal device (CyPass) for IOP control in open-angle glaucoma. Poster presented at: AAO Annual Meeting; October 18-19, 2010; Chicago, IL.
36. Craven ER, Khatana A, Hoeh H, et al. Minimally invasive, ab interno suprachoroidal micro-stent for IOP reduction in combination with phaco cataract surgery. Poster presented at: AAO Annual Meeting; October 2011; Orlando, FL.
37. Garcia-Feijoo J. Safety and efficacy of CyPass Micro-Stent as a stand-alone treatment for open-angle glaucoma: Wordwide clinical experience. Presented at: European Society of Cataract and Refractive Surgeons; 2012; Milan, Italy.
38. Hoeh H. Clinical outcomes of combined cataract surgery andimplantation of the CyPass Micro-Stent for the treatment of open-angle glaucma. Presented at: European Society of Cataract and Refractive Surgeons; 2012; Milan, Italy.
39. Grisanti S, Garcia-Feijoo J, Nardi M, et al. Minimally invasive ab-internosuprachoroidal micro-stent implantation (CyPass) for the primary treatment ofmedication-naïve patients with open angle glaucoma. Presented at: European Society of Cataract and Refractive Surgeons; 2012; Milan, Italy.

7

Ab Interno Stenting Procedures

Rohit Varma, MD

The traditional surgical approaches currently in use for the management of uncontrolled intraocular pressure (IOP) in patients with glaucoma include filtering surgery and aqueous shunt implantation. Trabeculectomy, currently the most commonly used drainage procedure, while effective, is plagued by significant visually impairing postoperative complications.[1-5] Another approach either as a primary procedure, or after trabeculectomy failure, is insertion of an aqueous shunt device such as an Ahmed or Baerveldt Implant. Aqueous shunt devices drain aqueous humor from the anterior chamber to a subconjunctival reservoir around a scleral fixated plate. Such devices, while effective, are also associated with significant postoperative complications and preclude future glaucoma surgery in the treated quadrant.[6-8]

A variety of new ab interno techniques are emerging that expand the surgical management of glaucoma. These new techniques have been referred to as MIGS.[9] While the main advantage of MIGS is that these procedures are less invasive and much safer, the primary therapeutic goal of the ab interno approaches is to provide similar efficacy as the traditional ab externo approaches (Figure 7-1).

Recently, Aquesys Inc (Aliso Viejo, CA) has developed a new ab interno subconjunctival procedure for lowering IOP in patients with glaucoma. The XEN Glaucoma Implant is made of cross-linked gelatin that is inserted using a minimally invasive ab interno approach that provides outflow of aqueous from the anterior chamber to the subconjunctival space created. The resulting outflow is not like a traditional ab externo trabeculectomy bleb.

The XEN Glaucoma Implant

The XEN Glaucoma Implant is a cylindrical implant composed of a porcine gelatin and cross-linked with glutaraldehyde. It is 6-mm long and varies in its internal diameter depending on the model. Details of the 3 models are presented in Figure 7-2. During the implantation procedure, the implant hydrates and swells in place to become a soft, nonmigrating drainage channel that is tissue conforming. The implant is collagen derived and cross-linked to become a permanent gelatin that provides a variety of desirable characteristics to the implant. The material has an extensive track record for medical use in a variety of geographic regions, including the European Union, the

Kahook MY.
MIGS: Advances in Glaucoma Surgery (pp 57-66).

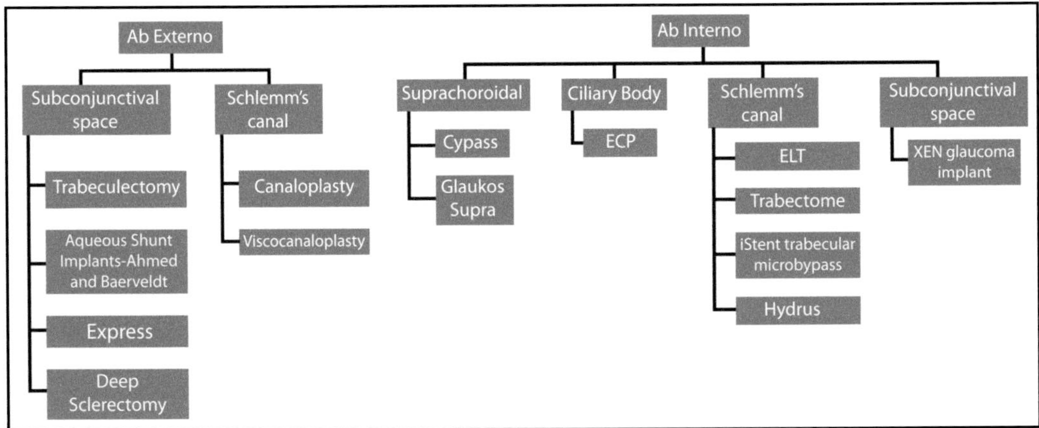

Figure 7-1. Glaucoma surgery: current technologies.

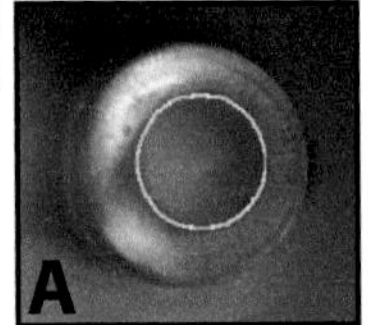

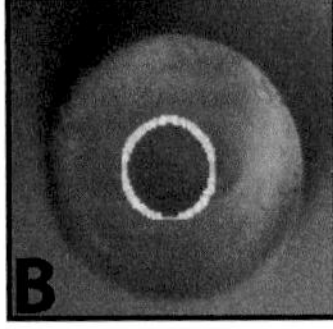

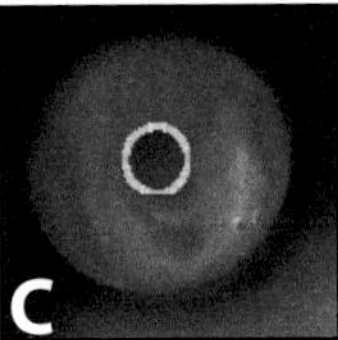

Figure 7-2. (A) XEN Glaucoma Implant. (B) XEN Mini Glaucoma Implant. (C) XEN Nano Glaucoma Implant.

United States, Asia, Australia, and Canada. The XEN Glaucoma Implant is made with gelatin that meets the compendial requirements of the European Pharmacopeia. The biocompatibility properties of gelatin are well established. Early clinical trials also show a remarkable lack of foreign body reactions in the human eye.

The implant reduces IOP by creating a permanent patent outflow pathway from the anterior chamber to the subconjunctival space through which the aqueous humor can flow. From the subconjunctival space, the aqueous humor has numerous potential drainage pathways, including diffusion through the conjunctiva, diffusion into the venous system of the sclera and conjunctiva, as well as potential lymphatic pathways.

The XEN Glaucoma Implant was designed as a solution to provide several key advantages over traditional glaucoma procedures:

- Minimally invasive ab interno procedure that reduces conjunctival incisions and subconjunctival and scleral dissection thereby reducing postoperative inflammation and scarring.
- In addition to reducing inflammation and scarring, the minimally invasive approach also allows multiple and repeatable implantations if needed over the lifetime of the patient.
- The implant shunts aqueous from the anterior chamber to subconjunctival space thus bypassing the trabecular meshwork, juxtacanalicular tissue, and Schlemm's canal. This eliminates the risk of reducing the efficacy of the implant due to any other outflow obstruction in the eye.
- Low and diffuse outflow into intact tissue anatomy and intact drainage pathways in the conjunctiva, giving maximum efficacy pressure reduction.

The laminar flow through a tube is calculated using the Hagen–Poiseuille equation, creating 3 different versions of implants:

$$\Phi = \frac{dV}{dt} = \upsilon \pi R^2 = \frac{\pi R^4}{8\eta}\left(\frac{-\Delta P}{\Delta x}\right) = \frac{\pi R^4}{8\eta}\frac{|\Delta P|}{L}$$

The 3 different versions were designed to accommodate the needs of different levels of IOP control (Figures 7-3 and 7-4). XEN has the largest inner diameter and will allow more flow for those

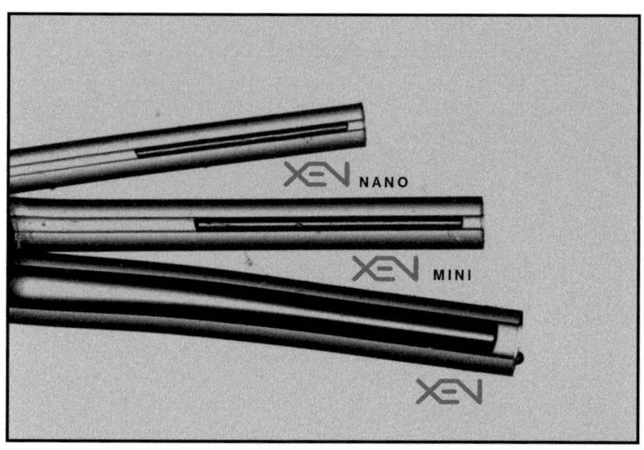

Figure 7-3. Microscopic pictures from a side view of implant versions with water column present at inner lumen.

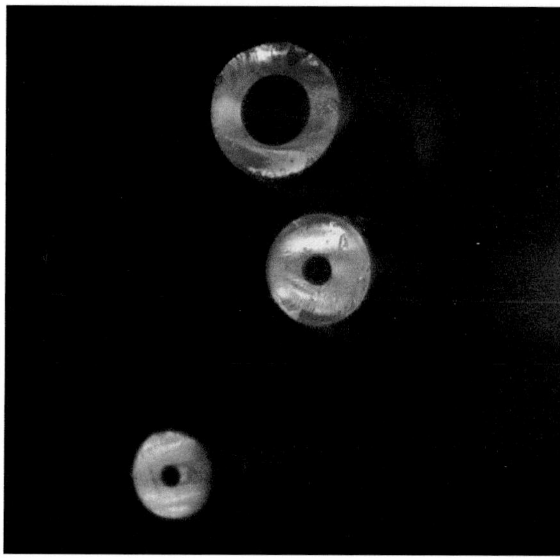

Figure 7-4. Microscopic picture from a cross-sectional view of implants.

patients who need maximal IOP lowering particularly if the patient has advanced optic nerve head damage. XEN Mini has a smaller lumen and is intended for patients who need moderate IOP lowering, and the XEN Nano has the smallest lumen, which is intended for patients with less advanced disease or ocular hypertension who are unable to tolerate or be controlled with topical medications (in which very minimal surgical risks are taken).

The 6-mm long implant is designed to be positioned with approximately 2 mm in the subconjunctival space, 3 mm intrascleral, and 1 mm in the anterior chamber. While achieving these suggested placement dimension parameters is ideal, it is not critical and makes this procedure a forgiving surgical procedure.

Procedure

The implantation is performed via an ab interno approach. The ab interno surgical approach is less invasive and preserves the integrity of the patient's conjunctiva, thereby preserving the patient's natural drainage pathways and reducing fibrosis and scarring.

The needle of the XEN Inserter (Figure 7-5) is designed to be minimally invasive by utilizing a small 25- or 27-gauge needle. The inserter (Figure 7-6) is designed to both protect the XEN Glaucoma Implant and to accurately place the implant into the correct anatomical location (it

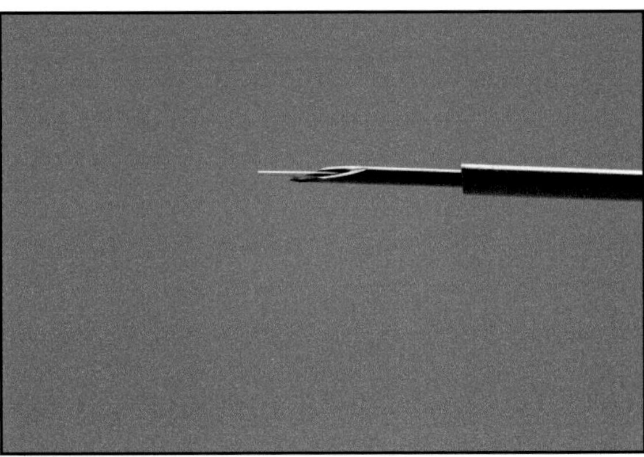

Figure 7-5. Close up picture of XEN Inserter showing the implant, needle, and sleeve (from left to right).

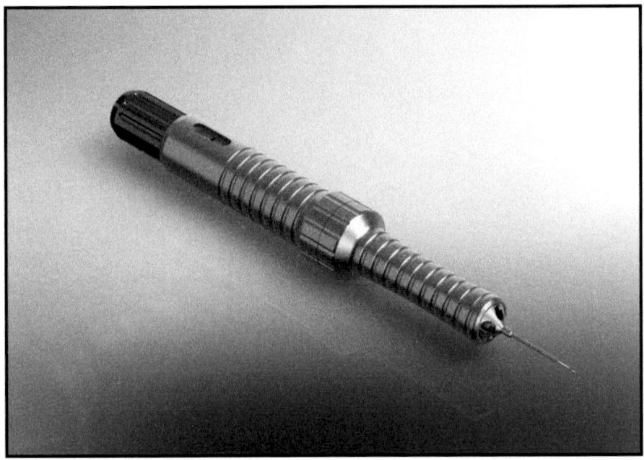

Figure 7-6. Picture of the XEN Inserter.

should be extended partially into the anterior chamber, through the angle and sclera, and exit into the subconjunctival space approximately 2.5 to 3.5 mm posterior to the limbus).

After standard ophthalmic preparation, the preloaded/single-use inserter is provided to the physician, individually packaged and sterile. To achieve the ideal intrascleral length of 3 mm, the surgeon should consider entering the peripheral cornea of the patient and direct the needle across the anterior chamber to the angle (Figure 7-7). Contrary to certain MIGS procedures where a specific target in the angle must be achieved, the entry zone of the angle is a broad and forgiving area, giving flexibility to use gonioscopy or not during the procedure. The needle can enter the angle anywhere from the Schwalbe's line to the scleral spur. Then the needle is guided through the sclera and into the subconjunctival space, creating a slit as it cuts through the scleral tissue.

As the needle bevel exits the sclera about 3 mm behind the limbus, the bevel angle is close to parallel with the conjunctiva tissue. This leads to the Tenon's and conjunctiva layers above the needle bevel to be pushed up versus being engaged in a penetrating fashion. As a result, perforating the conjunctiva with the needle bevel coming out of the sclera can be easily and consistently avoided. The surgeon is then able to directly visualize the entire needle's bevel in the subconjunctival space (Figure 7-8).

The physician then deploys the XEN Glaucoma Implant similar to an intraocular lens (IOL) insertion procedure. During this step, the implant is slowly deployed into position by the internal mechanism of the implanter (Figure 7-9). The procedure is then complete and the needle is fully withdrawn into a sleeve and the surgeon simply removes this blunt sleeve from the patient's eye (Figure 7-10). When the implant is in place, it immediately allows aqueous to travel from the anterior chamber to the subconjunctival space, bypassing the trabecular meshwork, Schlemm's canal, and the obstructed collector channels.

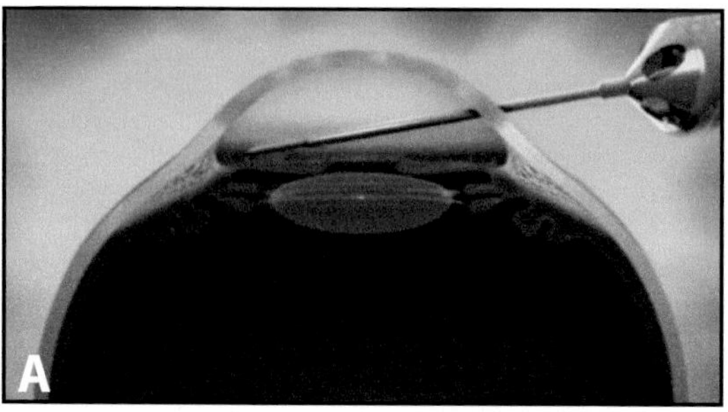

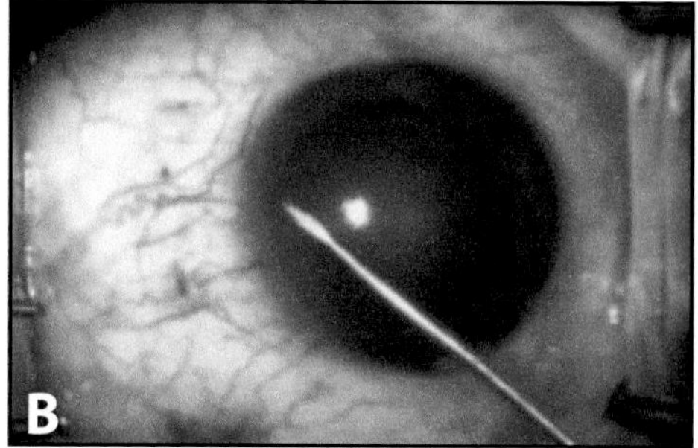

Figure 7-7. (A) Illustration (sagittal view) and (B) surgical picture of inserter passing across the anterior chamber to reach the angle.

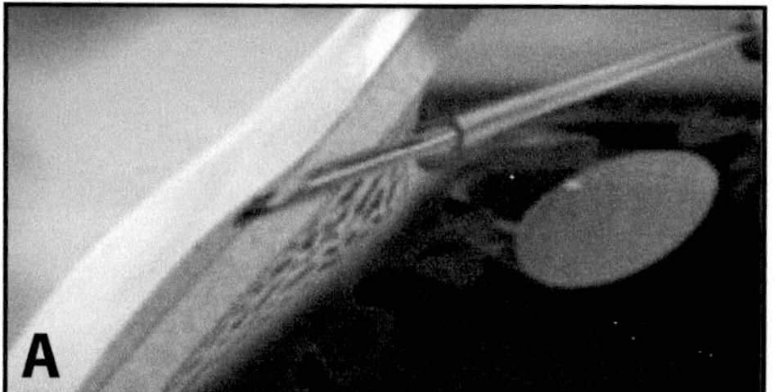

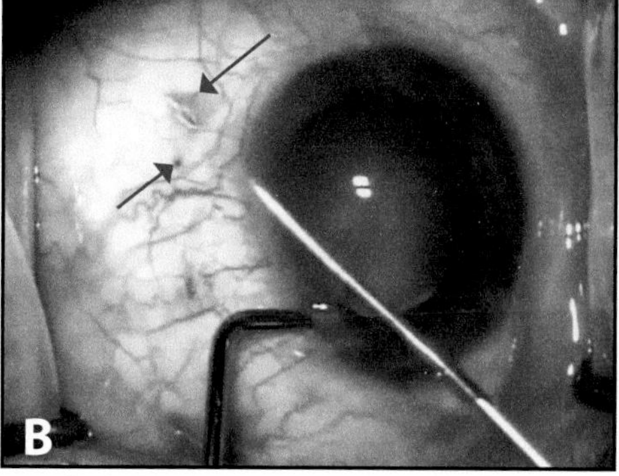

Figure 7-8. (A) Animation (sagittal view) and (B) surgical picture of needle entering the angle and creating a ~3-mm scleral tunnel (gonioless approach). Blue arrows pointing the premarked target exit at 3 mm from the limbus.

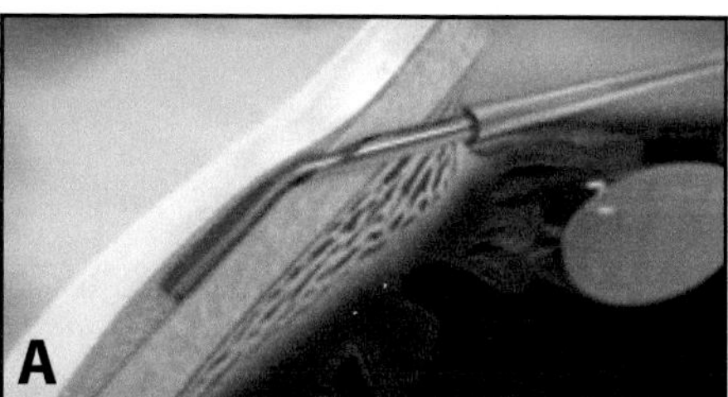

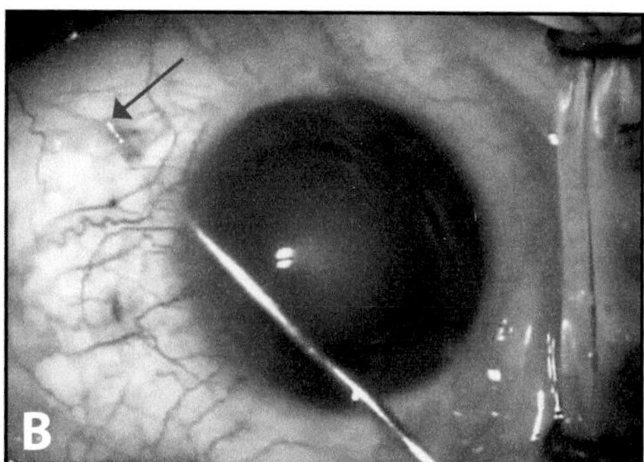

Figure 7-9. (A) Illustration (sagittal view) and (B) surgical picture of implant being deployed in position (blue arrow pointing at distal end of implant)

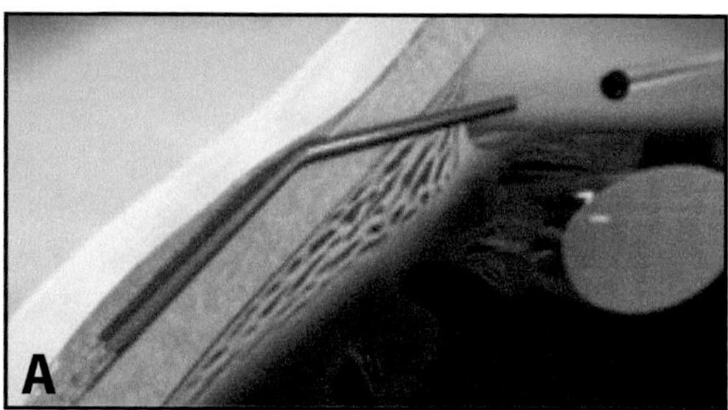

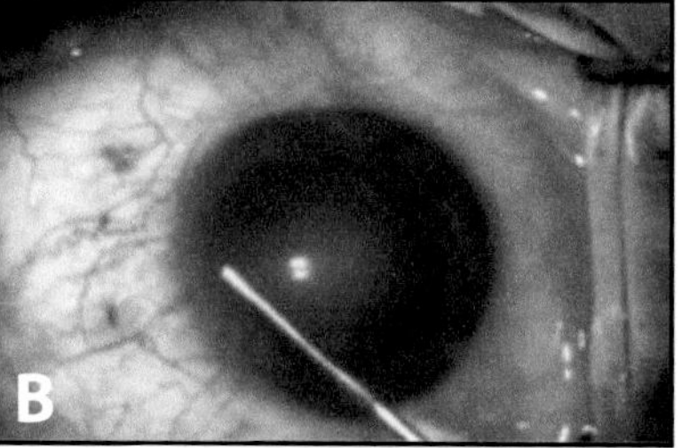

Figure 7-10. (A) Illustration (sagittal view) and (B) surgical picture of blunt sleeve being removed from eye.

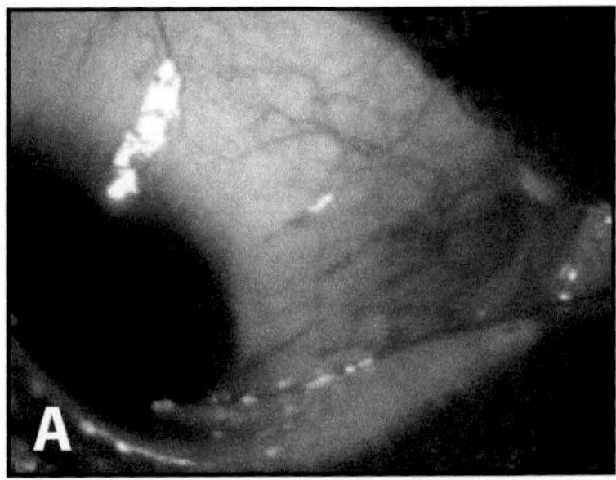

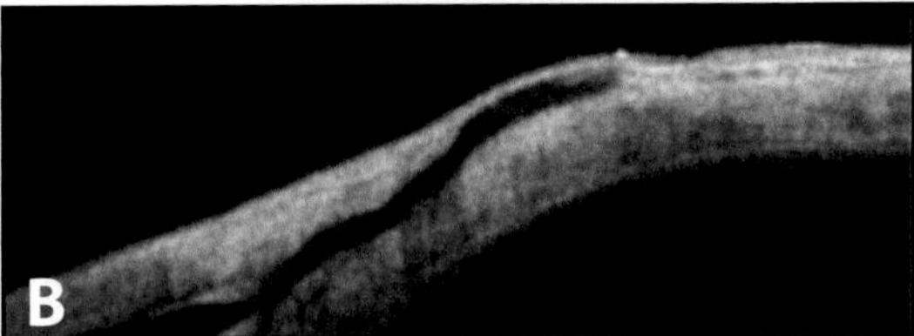

Figure 7-11. (A) Slit lamp picture and (B) OCT image of XEN Glaucoma Implant at 12 months postoperative. Bleb appearance is diffuse and low lying. Patient's IOP is 14 mm Hg on one prostaglandin. (Reprinted with permission from Iqbal Ike Ahmed, MD.)

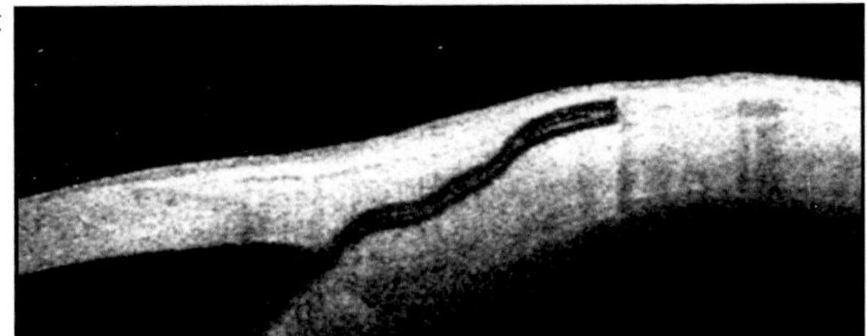

Figure 7-12. OCT image of XEN Glaucoma Implant and bleb at 3 months postoperative.

Mechanism of Action

As aqueous comes into contact with the XEN Glaucoma Implant, the gelatin material becomes hydrated, soft, and flexible and expands (by the time the implant is placed in the final position, this swelling process is mostly complete). The expansion of the outer wall of the implant (as shown in Figure 7-2) in combination with the elastic nature of the tissue separated by the needle, holds the implant in position once the needle has been removed from the eye. The subconjunctival flow is confirmed upon implantation. Initially the outflow can be medium in height but over the course of the first week, this outflow gradually reduces in volume as drainage pathways form from the subconjunctival space to the various outflow channels.[10]

Due to the dimensions and mechanical attributes of the implant material, a gentle and diffuse dispersion of aqueous into the nondissected Tenon's and subconjunctival space makes the morphology of an established, functioning outflow created by the XEN Glaucoma Implant different from the blebs seen after filtering surgeries. Long-term XEN outflow is predominately low lying and diffuse with moderate extension (Figure 7-11).

Initial studies using Visante AS-OCT images (N. Shoham-Hanzon, unpublished data, August 2012) to analyze the outflow demonstrate qualitative changes in outflow structure after XEN implantation. Conjunctival thickening was associated with reduction in IOP, as well as outflow wall thickness; however, not exclusively, as lower lying outflow, which was more diffuse, also showed good IOP reduction (Figure 7-12). In the majority of eyes, the OCT images showed a hyporeflective space between the conjunctiva and the sclera and indicated good filtration. The presence of microcysts throughout the epithelium (Figure 7-13) adds further anatomic evidence to the fact that the aqueous humor moves transconjunctivally after filtration surgery, following the

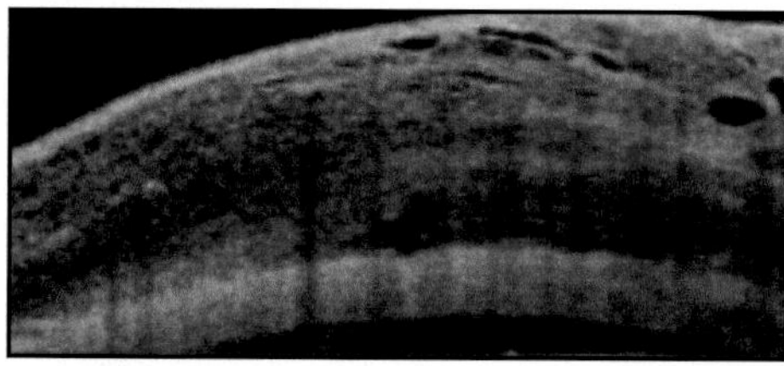

Figure 7-13. OCT image of bleb with microcysts present at one day postoperative after XEN implantation (nondissected conjunctiva).

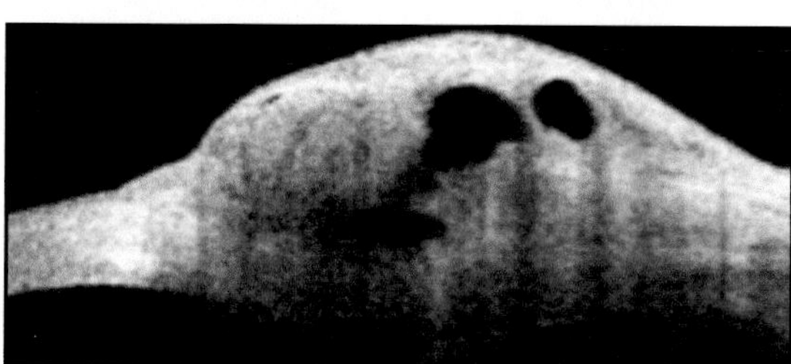

Figure 7-14. OCT image of bleb after EX-PRESS surgery.

mechanism of filtration.[11-17] This might indicate a more diffuse, controlled manner of outflow through the XEN Glaucoma Implant over a trabeculectomy or an EX-PRESS device (Figure 7-14).

In the majority of cases, the implant has been shown to provide long-term IOP lowering without the use of antimetabolites, such as MMC, at the time of surgery. In some cases of patients with high risk factors, such as previous history of fibrosis (eg, refractory cases or when an incisional surgery has failed already), a postoperative outflow enhancement procedure using antimetabolites is suggested to improve the long-term performance. This ability to tune the implant performance in the postoperative phase is another benefit of the XEN procedure. Early glaucoma patients without a long history of glaucoma drug usage showed remarkable low fibrosis rates and great long-term performances without any use of antimetabolites.

The mechanism of action of the XEN Glaucoma Implant procedure is consistent with other filtering procedures for glaucoma such as trabeculectomy and tube shunts, which bypass the traditional obstruction to outflow. The XEN Glaucoma Implant maintains a permanent patent outflow pathway between the anterior chamber and the subconjunctival space with a very soft, pliable cross-linked gelatin, which molds itself to the intrascleral anatomy. This soft, cross-linked gelatin is also likely to have minimal impact on the corneal endothelium. Finally, there is no need to create an iridotomy.

Clinical Data

Over the course of 6 years, a research program in animals was conducted to evaluate the feasibility of implanting a cylindrical gelatin implant for the treatment of open-angle glaucoma. The studies initially were conducted by Professor Dao-Yi Yu, Centre for Ophthalmology and Visual Science, University of Western Australia Lions Eye Institute. The research involved several studies conducted on over 100 animals (rabbits and primates) with several hundred microfistula implantations. The overall objective of these studies was to demonstrate the safety and feasibility of the XEN Glaucoma Implant for the treatment of open-angle glaucoma, which was successfully accomplished.

Preclinical testing was performed to assess the implant performance and functionality using both bench testing and animal experiments. Initial safety and feasibility assessments were undertaken and a risk analysis was conducted to determine the areas of potential risk to the patients. The results of the risk assessment were used to formulate a thorough verification and validation test plan, including complete verification or validation of all product specifications, sterilization

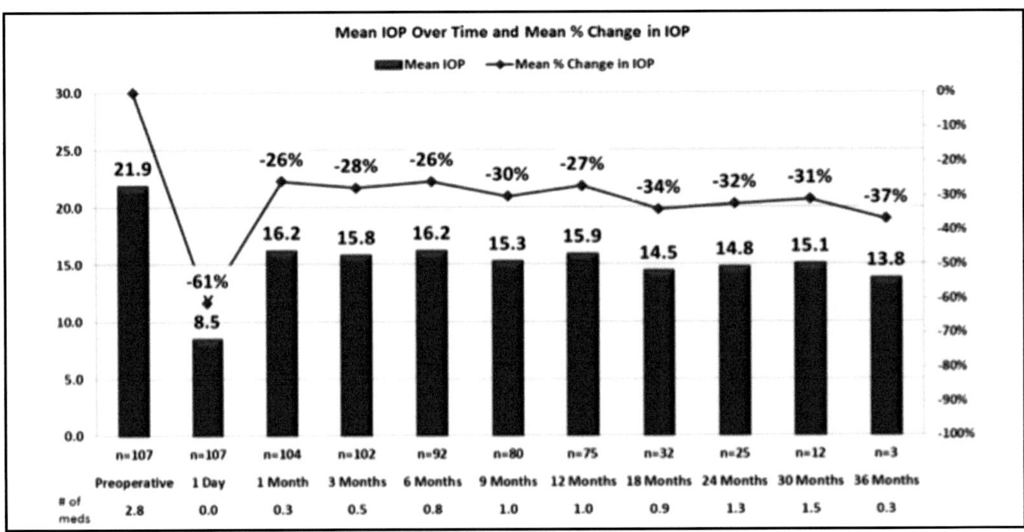

Figure 7-15. Current international clinical study results. *Mean preoperative IOP is best medicated. Patients were not washed out prior to surgery. **Antimetabolites were not used at the time of surgery.

validation, and biocompatibility testing. Extensive preclinical testing to confirm the safety and biocompatibility of the XEN Glaucoma Implant has been done.

Currently the XEN Glaucoma Implant is being studied in the United States and international trials where 107 subjects with primary open-angle glaucoma have been implanted (Figure 7-15). A multicenter (13 surgeons), prospective, nonrandomized, open-label clinical study is currently being held, with the purpose to evaluate the safety and effectiveness of the XEN Glaucoma Implant in reducing IOP in subjects with mild, moderate, and severe open-angle glaucoma, with a follow-up of up to 3 years.

The study enrollment and follow-up is still ongoing in multiple countries, and these results were collected during product development and learning curve phases.

From the 107 patients, 31 patients had XEN implanted at the beginning or at the end of cataract surgery and 76 patients had XEN implantation alone (30 patients had refractory glaucoma). As shown in Figure 7-15, the mean preoperative IOP was 21.9 mm Hg and mean postoperative IOPs were 15.9 mm Hg at 12 months, 14.5 at 18 months, and 14.8 at 24 months. This translates to a mean decrease in IOP (mm Hg) of –7.6 mm Hg (–34% reduction from best medicated IOP) at 18 months, and –7.5 mm Hg (–32% reduction from best medicated IOP) at 24 months. At 24 months, the number of antiglaucomatous medications were reduced by 54% (from a median of 3 medications to a median of one medication).

Conclusion

The XEN Glaucoma Implant is made with a known gelatin that is extremely well tolerated by the human body and has been shown to have a noninflammatory response. The softness of the material allows the device to be tissue conforming, which minimizes many of the problems associated with synthetic materials (eg, migration, erosion, endothelial cell damage). Importantly, the XEN Glaucoma Implant is an effective surgical approach to access a well-known outflow path in the subconjunctival space. It was designed as a technology to provide a minimally invasive ab interno procedure while safely and significantly lowering the IOP of patients with early, moderate, advanced, and refractory glaucoma (Figures 7-16 to 7-18). Upon implantation, the device is designed to create a diffuse outflow of aqueous into the nondissected conjunctiva and untouched

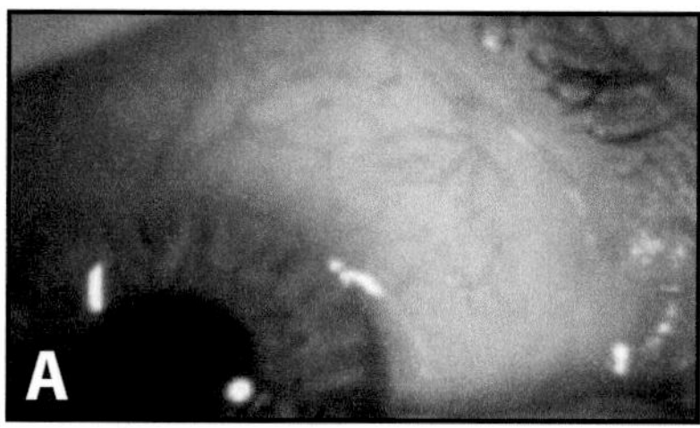

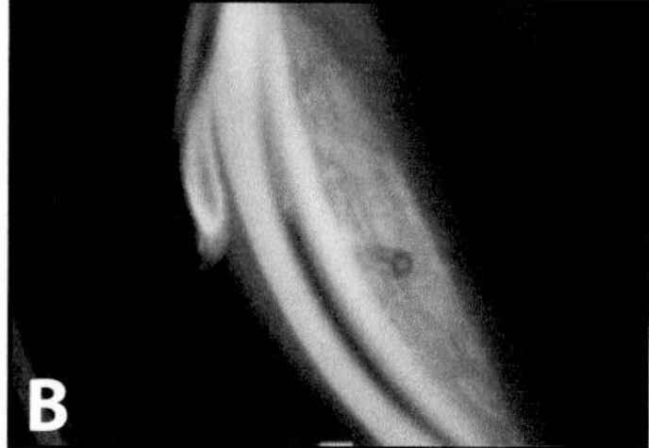

Figure 7-16. (A) Slit lamp picture and (B) gonioscopic view of eye at 12-month postoperative visit.

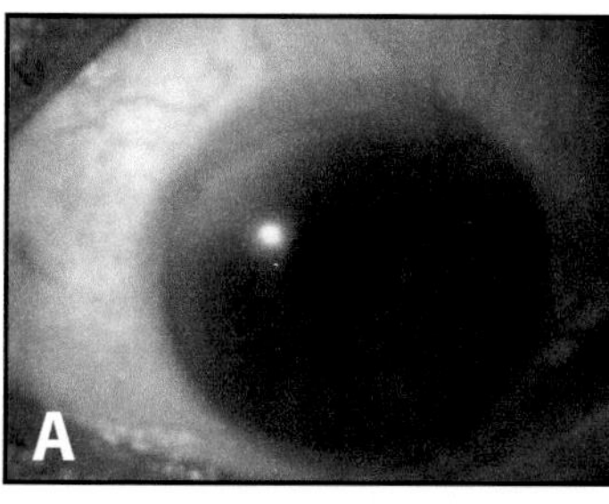

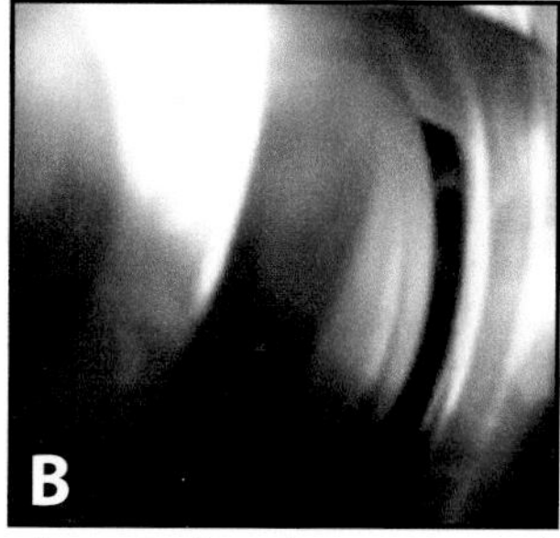

Figure 7-17. (A) Slit lamp picture and (B) gonioscopic view of eye at 12-month postoperative visit. Superonasal XEN Glaucoma Implant was implanted.

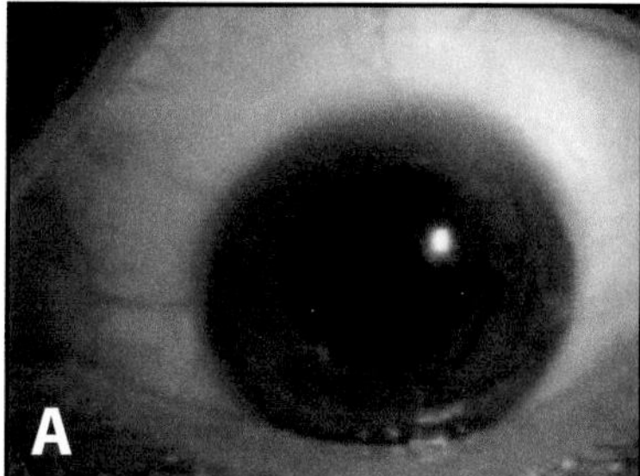

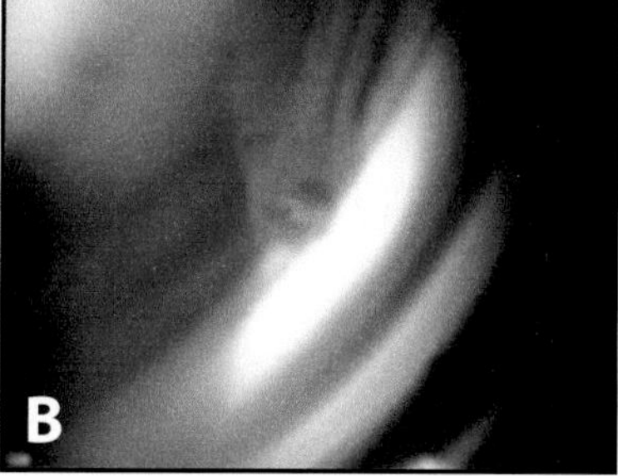

Figure 7-18. (A) Slit lamp picture and (B) gonioscopic view of eye at 12-month postoperative visit. Superonasal XEN Glaucoma Implant was implanted.

space. This conjunctiva-sparing ab interno approach allows an additional benefit where additional XEN Glaucoma Implants could be placed later on during the patient's lifetime, giving ophthalmologists a tool to adjust over the course of the patient's disease to different target IOP needs (Nano, Mini, and XEN).

References

1. Watson PG, Jakeman C, Ozturk M, Barnett MF, Barnett F, Khaw KT. Complications of trabeculectomy (a 20-year follow-up). *Eye (Lond).* 1990;4:425-438.
2. Nouri-Mahdavi K, Brigatti L, Weitzman M, Caprioli J. Outcomes of trabeculectomy for primary open-angle glaucoma. *Ophthalmology.* 1995;102:1760-1769.
3. Ticho U, Ophir A. Late complications after glaucoma filtering surgery with adjunctive 5-fluorouracil. *Am J Ophthalmol.* 1993;115:506-510.
4. Costa VP, Wilson RP, Moster M, Schmidt CM, Gandham S. Hypotony maculopathy following the use of topical mitomycin C in glaucoma filtration surgery. *Ophthalmic Surg.* 1993;24:389-394.
5. Ticho U, Ophir A. Late complications after glaucoma filtering surgery with adjunctive 5-fluorouracil. *Am J Ophthalmol.* 1993;115:506-510.

6. Topouzis F, Coleman AL, Choplin N, Bethlem MM, Hill R, Yu F, Panek WC, Wilson MR. Follow-up of the original cohort with the Ahmed glaucoma valve implant. *Am J Ophthalmol.* 1999;128:198-204.
7. Smith SL, Starita RJ, Fellman RL, Lynn JR. Early clinical experience with the Baerveldt 350-mm glaucoma implant and associated extraocular muscle imbalance. *Ophthalmology.* 1993;100:914-918.
8. Topouzis F, Yu F, Coleman AL. Factors associated with elevated rates of adverse outcome after cyclodestructive procedures versus drainage device procedures. *Ophthalmology.* 1998;105:2276-2281.
9. Francis BA, Singh K, Lin SC, Hodapp E, Jampel HD, Samples JR, Smith SD. Novel Glaucoma Procedures. A Report by the American Academy of Ophthalmology. *Ophthalmology.* 2011;118:1466–1480.
10. Dao-Yi Y et al. The critical role of the conjunctiva in glaucoma filtration surgery. *Prog Ret Eye Res.* 2009;28:303-328.
11. Addicks EM, Quigley HA, Green WR, et al. Histologic characteristics of filtering blebs in glaucomatous eyes. *Arch Ophthalmol.* 1983:101:795-798.
12. Labbé A, Dupas B, Hamard P, Baudouin C. In vivo confocal microscopy study of blebs after filtering surgery. *Ophthalmology.* 2005;112:1979-1986.
13. Guthoff R, Klink T, Schlunck, Grehn F. In vivo confocal microscopy of failing and functioning filtering blebs: Results and clinical correlations. *J Glaucoma.* 2006;15:552-8.
14. Messer EM, Zapp DM, Mackert MJ, et al. In vivo confocal microscopy of filtering blebs after trabeculectomy. *Arch Ophthalmol.* 2006;124:1095-1103.
15. Schmitt JM, Knüttel K, Yadlowsky M, Eckhaus MA. Optical-coherence tomography of a dense tissue: statistics of attenuationand backscattering. *Phys Med Biol.* 39:1994;1705-1720.
16. Picht G, Grehn F. Sickekissenentwicklung nach trabekulektomien. *Ophthalmologe.* 1998:95;380-387.
17. Singh M, Chew PTK, Friedman DS, et al. Imaging of trabeculaectomy blebs using anterior segment optical coherence tomography. *Ophthalmology.* 2007;114:47-53.

8

Ab Interno Trabeculectomy (Trabectome)

Mina B. Pantcheva, MD and Leonard K. Seibold, MD

Ab interno trabeculectomy with the Trabectome (NeoMedix Corporation, Tustin, CA) is a minimally invasive glaucoma surgery used to decrease the intraocular pressure (IOP) by specifically removing and ablating a segment of the trabecular meshwork (TM) and the inner wall of Schlemm's canal (SC). The Trabectome was introduced in the United States in early 2004, when the FDA approved the device for treatment of adult and juvenile open-angle glaucoma. The scientific rationale for the Trabectome is based on the concept that one of the main sites of resistance to aqueous outflow is the TM and the inner wall of SC. Thus, removing these structures effectively bypasses the resistance, improves aqueous outflow, and reduces the IOP. The IOP in treated eyes would then theoretically depend on the pressure in the collector channels and the episcleral venous pressure (EVP).

Barkan developed the earliest technique to increase outflow through SC by incising the TM and exposing SC to the anterior chamber directly.[1] This has been very successful in cases of congenital or infantile glaucoma, but the results in adults with primary open-angle glaucoma (POAG) have been disappointing. The presumed higher elasticity of the trabecular tissues in infants may allow the cut ends of the TM to retract, preventing their reapproximation and closure from fibrosis.[2] The adult angle tissue contains thicker trabecular beams with less elastic tissue morphologically. This may explain why the severed ends of TM after goniotomy in adults are more likely to fold back into their original position with scar formation across the incision.[3,4] Complete excision or ablation of the TM would, in theory, decrease the likelihood of reapproximation and thereby reduce the possibility for failure. The Trabectome system is thought to selectively remove the TM and possibly promote some retraction of the incision edges by cauterization. The Trabectome procedure spares the conjunctiva and does not result in bleb formation. Thus, if adequate long-term IOP control is not achieved, future incisional glaucoma surgery remains an option. Long-term success of this device is still unclear, and more data are needed to understand the full role of this technique in the surgical management of glaucoma. Potential disadvantages are the lack of circumferential flow in SC (limiting outflow to the collector channels exposed by the area of treatment), the potential for cleft closure, and the limitation of IOP reduction by EVP and collector channel resistance.

Kahook MY.
MIGS: Advances in Glaucoma Surgery (pp 67-75).

Device Design

The device concept was to provide a safe method to permanently ablate a segment of the TM and SC inner wall while avoiding closure of the created cleft from fibrosis and without causing damage to surrounding tissue. The device was to be used with standard anterior segment surgical techniques and equipment from an ab interno approach.

The Trabectome device consists of a disposable handpiece with a 19.5-gauge tip that will fit through a 1.6-mm corneal incision. The handpiece is connected to a console with irrigation and aspiration in addition to a simple electrocautery generator. The foot pedal controls the irrigation, aspiration, and electrocautery ablation via a stepwise foot control similar to modern phacoemulsification systems. The tip of the handpiece is specially designed with an insulated footplate that is pointed for ease of insertion through the TM into SC. The footplate protects the underlying tissues to preserve normal downstream aqueous outflow and is coated with a proprietary multilayered polymer, which provides exceptional thermal stability, mechanical strength, biocompatibility, and chemical resistance in laboratory testing. The aspiration port is in close proximity (approximately 0.3 mm) to the cautery electrode, and serves to remove debris during ablation. The irrigation port is positioned 3 mm from the surgical site and serves the dual purpose of keeping the eye pressurized and dissipating heat energy.

Although the irrigation and aspiration system's role is important, the high-frequency electrocautery generator is the pivotal point of this technology. The generator is a modified 800-EU unit from Aaron/Bovie (St. Petersburg, FL), and operates at a frequency of 550 kHz with adjustable power setting in 0.1-watt increments up to 10 watts (recommended range 0.5 to 1.5 W). The target tissue is disrupted and disintegrated by applying heat energy in bursts with a high peak power and low duty cycle. This ablation approach equates to high-energy bursts, which are bunched into small increments with comparably long time intervals in between. As a result, disruption and disintegration of tissue is theoretically achieved rather than a thermal-coagulation effect such as that seen in traditional cautery of blood vessels.[5,6] However, there have been reports illustrating thermal damage with this device.[7]

Procedure

In preparation for the procedure, after the area is prepped and draped, the patient's head is rotated opposite the eye receiving treatment and the microscope is tilted to allow a direct gonioscopic view of the angle. A 1.6-mm clear corneal incision is made near the limbus temporally and angled parallel to the iris. Viscoelastic is injected to deepen the angle and stabilize the anterior chamber. The Trabectome handpiece (Figure 8-1) is advanced nasally across the anterior chamber with the infusion on. A modified Swan-Jacobs gonioscopy lens is used to visualize the target TM nasally as the instrument tip is advanced across the anterior chamber. The tip of the footplate is gently inserted through the TM into SC as is customary with goniotomy procedures. A foot switch activates the irrigation, aspiration, and electro-surgical elements that ablate and remove the strip of TM and inner wall of SC as the surgeon slowly advances the instrument (Figure 8-2). The treatment is carried out along the meshwork in either a clockwise or counterclockwise direction using the insertion site as a fulcrum. A strip of TM and SC tissue spanning 90 to 120 degrees is typically ablated and removed during treatment. This may be accomplished in a single continuous circular movement under direct gonioscopic visualization or in 2 interrupted motions extending both clockwise and counterclockwise from the nasal starting point 180 degrees away from the incision. Intraoperative reflux of blood through the resulting cleft is often encountered and considered desirable as this usually confirms appropriate ab interno "unroofing" of SC. The initial power setting of 0.7 to 0.8 W is titrated up or down as needed depending on the result desired. If charring of

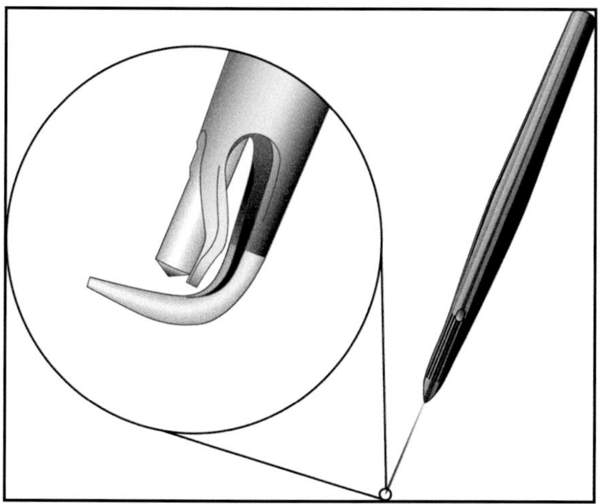

Figure 8-1. Trabectome handpiece and tip showing the footplate, which is designed to protect surrounding tissues from thermal damage.

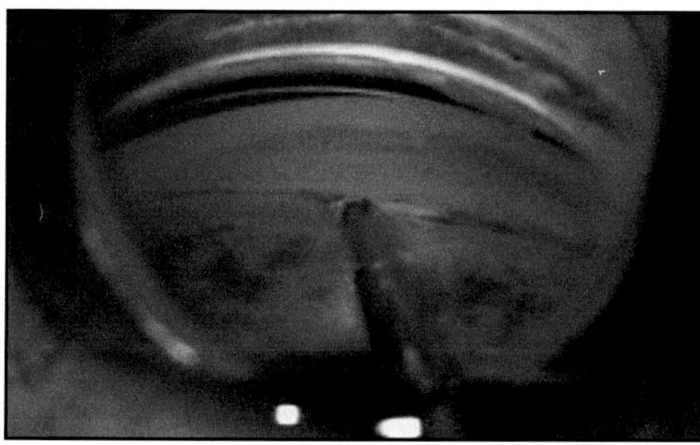

Figure 8-2. Intraoperative photo of trabectome treatment showing removal of TM (to the right of the probe) with the tip advancing from right to left.

tissue is noted, the power should be turned down, while a higher power setting may be needed to ablate a wider strip of TM. A thorough aspiration of the viscoelastic is performed and the incision is closed with a 10-0 nylon suture.

Preclinical Studies

Francis et al performed a histopathologic analysis to confirm the ability of the Trabectome device to remove the target tissue and to compare it with simulated goniotomy.[5] This in vitro analysis was performed on fresh donor human corneoscleral rims. Each complete rim was divided into 3 segments, each of which was used for either (1) control, (2) Maumenee goniotomy knife (Bausch & Lomb Surgical, Rochester, NY) incision, or (3) Trabectome application. Various power settings ranging from 0.3 to 5.0 W were used to assess the effects of the ablation on the surrounding tissue.

Two specimens underwent simulated goniotomy. One of them displayed disruption of the TM with no apparent separation of the TM due to the anterior and posterior segments of TM overlapping. The other specimen was shown to have a large separation between the severed ends of the TM; however, this was accompanied by a large incision into the sclera deep to SC. Of the 20 specimens treated with the Trabectome system, 4 specimens showed no separation of the TM. The authors noted that the results in 2 of those appear to be due to surgical technique, with the instrument footplate failing to pass into SC. Thus, only 16 of 18 specimens undergoing appropriate treatment failed to show disruption of the TM with separation of the anterior and posterior margins. In these 18 samples the mean separation was 130.5 μm. There was no evidence of thermal damage deep to the TM or in the surrounding tissues in any of the tissue samples. Coagulation was observed in 10 of 20 treated samples, affecting the anterior TM more than the posterior TM. There was no difference in the size of the openings in the TM, the presence of coagulative damage of the TM, or the damage to surrounding structures with respect to the ablation power settings (0.3 to 5.0 W). However, the sample size at each power setting was small and variable. Several of the donors were young and there could be age-related changes to the TM that may affect the retraction of the tissue. Because of the small sample size and the different number of samples in each group, no significant trend could be found with respect to the age of the donor rim.

Clinical Studies

The initial clinical report of ab interno trabeculectomy with the Trabectome included 37 patients with a follow-up ranging between 3 months (n = 37) and 13 months (n = 11). Mean IOP reduction of about 38% was achieved at the 6-month follow-up (n = 25).[8] The number of adjunctive medications decreased from 1.2 ± 0.6 among preoperative patients on medications (n = 34) to 0.4 ± 0.6 among all patients at 6 months (n = 25). Blood reflux was reported in all eyes upon instrument withdrawal at the conclusion of the surgery and cleared by slit lamp examination at a mean of 6.4 ± 4.1 days postoperatively. Other complications included peripheral anterior synechiae (24.3%), corneal injury (16.2%), focal iris adhesion to spur or posterior meshwork (13.5%), and pressure spike defined as postoperative IOP > 5 mm Hg above baseline (5.4%). In a subsequent larger series of Trabectome-treated patients (n = 101) with follow-up extended up to 30 months, the overall success rate, defined as IOP lower than 21 mm Hg with or without medication and no subsequent glaucoma surgery, was determined to be 84%.[9] Furthermore, a very low incidence of early hypotony and loss of vision in excess of 2 lines was reported with this procedure (< 1% for both parameters).

Filippopoulos and Rhee published a review reporting an interim analysis of an ongoing prospective multicenter study evaluating the efficacy and safety of this novel procedure.[10] The report described the clinical outcome of 679 consecutive patients undergoing ab interno trabeculectomy with the Trabectome with a maximum follow-up of up to 52 months. The average reduction in IOP was 29% at 6-months follow-up (n = 106), 34% at 12-months follow-up (n = 65), and 30% at 24-months follow-up (n = 30). The level of pressure reduction at 24 months (30%) was sustained in the few patients who reached 48-months follow-up (n = 13). In addition, a reduction in the number of glaucoma medications by approximately 2 medications was documented, which peaked at 10-months follow-up and remained stable thereafter. Very few patients (n = 7, 1%) experienced early transient hypotony (IOP < 5 mm Hg) at the first postoperative day. The most common and the only clinically significant complication was a spike in IOP (IOP > 21 mm Hg) in the early postoperative period (19.7%). The cumulative incidence of a subsequent glaucoma surgical procedure was 8% for this cohort with the overwhelming majority (85%) of surgeries being performed within 6 months after the Trabectome procedure, and 67% of the treating physicians preferring trabeculectomy as the second procedure. In 30% of the cases, the Trabectome procedure was combined with cataract extraction.

Francis et al reported the short-term results of combined phacoemulsification and ab interno trabeculectomy with the Trabectome (n = 304). In most cases, the ab interno trabeculectomy was performed first, followed by cataract extraction by phacoemulsification.[11] A successful outcome, defined as a 20% or greater drop in IOP or decrease in glaucoma medications without need for additional medications or glaucoma procedures, including laser trabeculoplasty, was achieved in 78% of patients at 6 months (n = 106) and 64% at 12 months (n = 34). Nine patients (3%) required secondary glaucoma procedures (7 trabeculectomy, 1 aqueous tube shunt, 1 selective laser trabeculoplasty). The glaucoma medications were reduced from 2.65 ± 1.13 before surgery to 1.44 ± 1.29 at 1 year after surgery. No patient had a decrease in Snellen visual acuity of 2 or more lines. An IOP spike of 10 mm Hg or greater occurred in 8.6% of patients 1 day postoperatively and in 2.0% by 1 week. There were no complications such as those seen after trabeculectomy with mitomycin C (MMC) (eg, sustained hypotony, choroidal effusion or hemorrhage, aqueous misdirection, infection, bleb formation, or wound leaks).

Minckler et al reported a retrospective case series of 1127 Trabectome surgeries, with 738 of them being Trabectome-only and 366 of them combined Trabectome-cataract surgeries.[12] The decrease in IOP among Trabectome-only cases with or without medications was 40% at 24 months (n = 46), 41% at 36 months (n = 35), and 35% at 60 months (n = 2). The mean preoperative IOP of 25.7 ± 7.7 mm Hg was decreased to 16.4 ± 4.5 mm Hg. In Trabectome-only cases (n = 738), Kaplan–Meier plots defining "failure" as IOP > 21 and not reduced by 20% below baseline (on 2 consecutive visits after 2 weeks follow-up) or subsequent surgery indicated a failure rate of approximately 35% at 24 months. When "failure" was defined as IOP > 21 or not reduced by 20% below baseline or subsequent surgery for the same group at the same time-point, the failure rate rose to approximately 55%. The mean decrease in adjunctive medications for Trabectome-only cases was from a preoperative mean of 2.9 ± 1.30 to a postoperative mean of 1.8 ± 1.4 antiglaucoma medications. Failure defined as additional glaucoma surgery occurred in 14% of the Trabectome-only cases. The mean IOP of patients who underwent a Trabectome-cataract procedure was 20.0 ± 6.2 mm Hg at baseline and dropped to 15.9 ± 3.3 mm Hg by 12 months after surgery (n = 45). The authors reported a reduction in medications from 2.63 ± 1.12 at baseline to 1.50 ± 1.36 at 12 months.

Based on the available clinical studies, ab interno trabeculectomy with the Trabectome appears to be a promising MIGS approach to lowering IOP when attempting to halt or slow down progression of IOP-induced glaucomatous optic neuropathy. It is relatively easy to perform, reproducible, has a low incidence of early postoperative hypotony (0% to 1%), and can provide adequate IOP control.[10] Furthermore, the conjunctiva remains undisturbed during this procedure, allowing conventional glaucoma surgery like trabeculectomy or glaucoma drainage implantation to still be available if better IOP control is needed. This was confirmed by Jea and colleagues' retrospective review comparing eyes undergoing trabeculectomy following Trabectome (n = 34) to eyes undergoing trabeculectomy as a primary procedure (n = 42).[13] They found no difference in IOP decrease and success rates between the 2 groups. The Trabectome procedure cannot be expected to achieve IOP levels lower than EVP once the TM has been removed. Thus, it is usually not suitable for patients with end-stage optic nerve cupping or low tension glaucoma who are in need of IOPs below the level of EVP.

Jea et al conducted a retrospective nonrandomized review comparing the effect of ab interno trabeculectomy (n = 115) with trabeculectomy (n = 102).[14] They used 4 definitions for failure/success. Definition 1 was IOP ≤ 21 mm Hg or ≥ 20% reduction below baseline on 2 consecutive follow-up visits after 1 month. Definition 2 was IOP ≤ 18 mm Hg or ≥ 30% reduction below baseline on 2 consecutive follow-up visits after 1 month. Definition 3 was IOP ≤ 21 mm Hg and definition 4 was IOP ≤ 18 mm Hg. All 4 definitions included the criteria of IOP ≤ 5 mm Hg on 2 consecutive follow-up visits after 1 month, additional glaucoma surgery, or loss of light perception vision. Secondary outcome measures included number of glaucoma medications and occurrence of complications. IOP decreased from 28.1 ± 8.6 mm Hg at baseline to 15.9 ± 4.5 mm Hg (43.5% reduction, range 9 to 19 mm Hg) at month 24 in the ab interno trabeculectomy group (AIT). In the trabeculectomy with MMC group, IOP decreased from 26.3 ± 10.9 mm Hg at baseline to 10.2 ± 4.1 mm Hg (61.3% reduction, range 6 to 18 mm Hg) at 24 months. The number of antiglaucoma medications was 3.3 ± 1.3 and 2.2 ± 1.6 at baseline and month 24, respectively, in the AIT group, and 3.4 ± 1.0 and 0.5 ± 1.0, respectively, in the trabeculectomy with MMC group. The success rates at 1 year postoperatively using failure definition 1 were 36.1% and 85.6% in the AIT and trabeculectomy with MMC groups, respectively. The success rates at postoperative year 2 were significantly less in the AIT group regardless of failure definition used. Using definition 1, success rates were 22.4% and 76.1% in the AIT and trabeculectomy with MMC groups, respectively ($P < 0.001$). The success rates at 2 years postoperatively were 10.4% and 66.2% with definition 2,

43.0% and 76.3% with definition 3, and 25.7% and 73.7% with definition 4 in the AIT and trabeculectomy with MMC groups, respectively ($P < 0.001$).

With the exception of hyphema, the occurrence of postoperative complications was more frequent in the trabeculectomy group. Inadvertent creation of a cyclodialysis cleft in the AIT group occurred in one eye. Other complications, such as early and persistent hypotony (4.9%), wound leak, shallow anterior chamber, conjunctival buttonhole, corneal abrasion, and bullous keratopathy, occurred only in the trabeculectomy group. In the AIT group, the reasons for failure were the need for additional glaucoma surgery in 50 of 79 eyes (63.3% of failures) and inadequate IOP reduction in 29 eyes (36.7% of failures). Overall, the occurrence of additional procedures after AIT (43.5%) was significantly higher than in the trabeculectomy group (10.8%, $P < 0.001$).

Long-term data are expected to be available as well as randomized prospective studies against trabeculectomy or drainage implants to clarify the role for ab interno trabeculectomy with Trabectome in the management of patients with open-angle glaucoma.

Other Approaches to Ab Interno Trabeculectomy

Other manual devices have been developed to improve and further advance the ab interno trabeculectomy technique and outcomes. These instruments offer certain advantages over the more elaborate setup and disposable parts of the Trabectome. They are reusable and relatively inexpensive and can be added to a standard cataract surgical tray. In addition, they lack moving parts or the need for coupled irrigation or a separate power source allowing for inexpensive manufacturing and rapid acquisition of surgical expertise.

Goniocurettage

The underlying concept of goniocurettage is to bluntly remove rather than incise the TM. This allows the aqueous humour to either egress into SC or to seep out through microsplittings in the posterior scleral wall where the external wall of the canal is damaged.[15] The trabecular tissue is scraped away from the scleral sulcus using a device called the gonioscraper. The instrument has a small handle and a slightly convex arm for intraocular use and resembles a cyclodialysis spatula. However, the tip of the instrument is shaped like a miniature bowl, 300 µm in diameter, with sharpened edges. To abrade the TM in a clockwise and counter-clockwise fashion, the scoop is vertically angled at 90 degrees to either side.

The procedure is performed under direct visualization of the anterior chamber angle through an operating microscope using a surgical gonioscopy lens. Following injection of viscoelastic, the gonioscraper is inserted into the anterior chamber through a temporal clear corneal incision and directed against the TM on the opposite (nasal) side. The scraper is lightly passed over 2 to 3 clock hours to either side of the nasal circumference of the chamber angle. Great care is taken while peeling off the uveal meshwork to not traumatize adjacent intraocular structures, such as the corneal endothelium or the base of the iris. At the end of the procedure, the viscoelastic along with the abraded trabecular debris is removed by means of irrigation-aspiration.

Jacobi et al[15] showed histologically that in addition to the peeling of the TM, goniocurettage also caused damage to the intracanalicular septa and the endothelium of the external wall of SC, and in some instances a disruption along the posterior wall of SC. Flaps of uveal tissue, capable of returning to their predissection position, were not observed in the specimens. Scanning electron microscopy showed that the TM was pulled away from its attachments, leaving ragged structures of SC within the scleral sulcus, exposing bare sclera.

In a recent prospective, nonrandomized clinical trial, 25 eyes of 25 patients with uncontrolled chronic open-angle glaucoma that had undergone failed filtering procedures were treated by goniocurettage.[16] Overall success, defined as postoperative IOP of 19 mm Hg or less with one

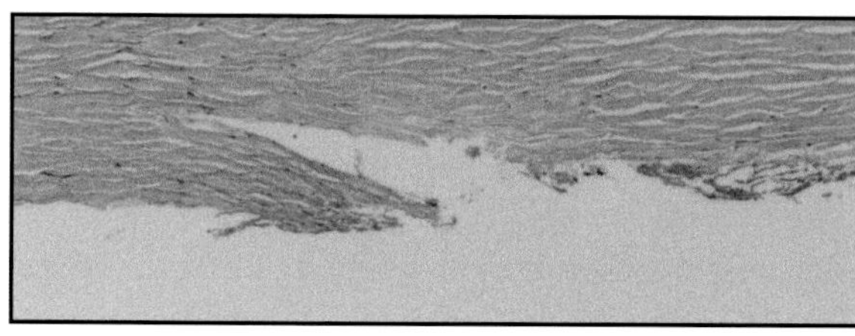

Figure 8-3. Post ab interno trabeculectomy with a novel dual-blade device illustrating removal of TM without surrounding damage to adjacent tissues.

pressure-reducing agent, was attained in 15 eyes (60%), with 5 eyes (20%) being controlled without medication. Follow-up averaged 32.6 ± 8.1 months (range, 30 to 45 months). Complications included localized Descemet's membrane detachment in 5 eyes (20%) and marked anterior chamber bleeding in 4 eyes (16%) due to perforations of prominent chamber angle vessels. Due to the sustained anterior chamber angle bleeding, the procedure was aborted in 2 eyes (8%). A reflux of blood from SC into the treatment area occurred in 22 eyes (88%) with no further sequelae. The postoperative IOP levels after goniocurettage remained in the high teens, even with medication with mean IOP of 17.7 ± 3.1 mm Hg (range, 10 to 19 mm Hg) at the final visit.

Larger sample data as well as randomized clinical studies against trabeculectomy or drainage implants are needed to clarify the role for this procedure in the management of patients with open-angle glaucoma.

Ab Interno Trabeculectomy Using a Novel Dual-Blade Device

Utilizing a new method for ab interno trabeculectomy, Dr. Malik Y. Kahook developed a novel dual-blade device for TM incision (see Chapter 3, Figure 3-6).[7] The size and tip of the blade allows for smooth entry into the SC, similar to techniques used for traditional goniotomy procedures. Once in place, the dual-blade tip is advanced through SC while the TM is elevated along a specially designed ramp that guides tissue toward a set of blades specifically positioned to incise and remove TM. In contrast to the Trabectome footplate, which is juxtaposed between the outer and the inner walls of the SC to provide protection during cautery, the dual-blade device transects TM and has a primary purpose of elevating TM off of the outer wall of SC. Elevating the TM along the ramp of the device as it moves forward leads to maximal tissue removal when incised by the superiorly placed and strategically angled dual blades. The excised TM may then be removed from the eye with forceps or aspirated during the irrigation/aspiration phase of viscoelastic removal. The angle between the distal cutting edge and the device handle is engineered to allow for maximal angle treatment through a single incision. The device geometry is designed to minimize any impact to adjacent tissues, such as Descemet's membrane, by leveraging specific angles between the handle and the distal blade as well as use of specific angles between the dual cutting blades and the adjacent cutting tip.

In vitro analysis was performed to evaluate the effects of this novel ab interno trabeculectomy device on 6 fresh donor human corneoscleral rims. The TM was incised using the (1) novel dual-blade device, (2) microvitreoretinal (MVR) blade (BD, Franklin Lakes, NJ), and (3) Trabectome. A total of 2 samples were used for each of the 3 treatment methods studied. Subsequently, human eye perfusion studies were performed to evaluate IOP-lowering effects of each device.

Histologic analysis showed that the MVR blade technique exhibited complete incision through the entire thickness of TM tissue. However, there was minimal removal of TM with large leaflets of tissue remaining and obvious blade injury to the adjacent deep sclera. Although the Trabectome also achieved an opening through the entirety of TM tissue into SC, leaflets of residual tissue still remained along with extensive charring from thermal injury. Tissue incised with the dual-blade device demonstrated a more complete removal of TM without collateral damage (Figure 8-3). All 3 treatment modalities achieved a significant reduction in measured IOP 30 minutes after treatment in the human eye perfusion model. Treatment with the dual-blade device and Trabectome resulted in a mean IOP reduction of 40% each, whereas the MVR blade achieved a 31% reduction. Although the percentage of IOP decrease was greater for Trabectome and the dual-blade device, there was no statistically significant difference in the IOP lowering between devices. There was no correlation between the number of degrees of TM treated and the percentage of IOP change for any device.

Future clinical studies are upcoming and needed to elucidate the safety and efficacy of the device compared to other reference devices.

Future Work

Emerging MIGS devices and procedures, such as Trabectome, raise certain questions that need to be addressed in order to provide for safe and consistent improvements in the management outcomes of our patients. One such question is whether bypassing the tissue with highest resistance in the conventional outflow pathway would be sufficient in all patients as the distal components of this pathway may also offer resistance. Kagemann et al noninvasively assessed the SC, collector channels, and intrascleral venous plexus using spectral domain ocular coherence tomography.[17] They found that the cross-sectional area of SC was larger at junctions with active collector channels and significantly larger on the nasal side than on the temporal, which is the most common site for canal-based surgery using clear corneal temporal incisions.

Provocative gonioscopy and channelography with a flexible microcatheter and fluorescein tracer during canaloplasty was used to assess the aqueous outflow pathway in 28 Black patients with POAG.[18] The level of IOP after surgery correlated with the grade of blood reflux and episcleral venous egress ($P < 0.001$). Such findings suggest that anatomical and functional assessment of conventional outflow structures distal to the TM can be valuable in predicting postoperative outcome. Further studies are needed to investigate the width of a TM incision, the number of devices to be inserted, and the length of a device to be used. Each of those parameters could be modified to achieve an optimal outflow increase.

The use of these devices will require improvement in angle visualization to achieve their correct placement and minimize complications. Future intraoperative gonioscopy techniques may include direct gonioscopy (without need for microscope or patient head tilt) and/or endoscopic visualization of the angle.

References

1. Barkan O. Technique of goniotomy for congenital glaucoma. *Arch Ophthalmol.* 1949; 41(1):65-82.
2. Horstmann HJ, Rohen JW, Sames K. Age-related changes in the composition of proteins in the trabecular meshwork of the human eye. *Mech Ageing Dev.* 1983;21(2):121-136.
3. McMenamin PG, Lee WR, Aitken DA. Age-related changes in the human outflow apparatus. *Ophthalmology.* 1986;93(2):194-209.
4. Hirano K, Kobayashi M, Kobayashi K, et al. Age-related changes of microfibrils in the cornea and trabecular meshwork of the human eye. *Jpn J Ophthalmol.* 1991;35(2):166-174.
5. Francis BA, See RF, Rao NA et al. Ab interno trabeculectomy: development of a novel device (Trabectome) and surgery for open-angle glaucoma. *J Glaucoma.* 2006;15(1):68-73.
6. Nguyen QH. Trabectome: A novel approach to angle surgery in the treatment of glaucoma. *Int Ophthalmol Clin.* 2008;48(4):65-72.
7. Seibold LK, SooHoo JR, Ammar DA, Kahook MY. Preclinical investigation of ab interno trabeculectomy using a novel dual-blade device. *Am J Ophthalmol.* 2013;155(3):524-529.e2.
8. Minckler DS, Baerveldt G, Alfaro MR, Francis BA. Clinical results with the Trabectome for treatment of open-angle glaucoma. *Ophthalmology.* 2005;112(6):962-978.
9. Minckler DS, Baerveldt G, Ramirez MA, Mosaed S et al. Clinical results with Trabectome, a novel surgical device for treatment of open-angle glaucoma. *Trans Am Ophthalmol Soc.* 2006;104:40-50.

10. Filippopoulos T, Rhee DJ. Novel surgical procedures in glaucoma: advances in penetrating glaucoma surgery. *Curr Opin Ophthalmol.* 2008;19(2):149-154.
11. Francis BA, Minckler D, Dustin L, Kawji S et al. Combined cataract extraction and trabeculotomy by the internal approach for coexisting cataract and open-angle glaucoma: initial results. *J Cataract Refract Surg.* 2008;34(7):1096-1103.
12. Minckler D, Mosaed S, Dustin L, et al. Trabectome (trabeculectomy-internal approach): additional experience and extended follow-up. *Trans Am Ophthalmol Soc.* 2008;106:149–159.
13. Jea SY, Mosaed S, Vold SD, Rhee DJ. Effect of a failed trabectome on subsequent trabeculectomy. *J Glaucoma.* 2012 Feb;21(2):71-75.
14. Jea SY, Francis BA, Vakili G, et al. Ab interno trabeculectomy versus trabeculectomy for open-angle glaucoma. *Ophthalmology.* 2012;119(1):36-42.
15. Jacobi PC, Dietlein TS, Krieglstein GK. Technique of goniocurettage: a potential treatment of advanced open-angle glaucoma. *Br J Ophthalmol.* 1997;8(4):302-307.
16. Jacobi PC, Dietlein TS, Krieglstein GK. Goniocurettage for removing trabecular meshwork: clinical results of a new surgical technique in advanced chronic open-angle glaucoma. *Am J Ophthalmol.* 1999;127(5):505-510.
17. Kagemann L, Wollstein G, Ishikawa H, et al. Identification and assessment of Schlemm's canal by spectral-domain optical coherence tomography. *Invest Ophthalmol Visual Sci.* 2010;51(8):4054–4059.
18. Grieshaber MC, Pienaar A, Olivier J, Stegmann R. Clinical evaluation of the aqueous outflow system in primary open-angle glaucoma for canaloplasty. *Invest Ophthalmol Visual Sci.* 2010; 51(3):1498–1504.

9

Endocyclophotocoagulation and Other Cyclodestructive Procedures

Mahmoud Khaimi, MD and Jacob W. Brubaker, MD

Endocyclophotocoagulation (ECP) has been available for over 15 years. It takes the principles used in transscleral cyclophotocoagulation (TSCPC) and couples the approach with endoscopic capabilities. TSCPC uses an external diode laser to ablate the ciliary body through the scleral wall. The 810-nm diode laser is ideal, as the melanin in the epithelium of the ciliary body preferentially absorbs this wavelength, leading to more targeted destruction. By ablating and destroying portions of the ciliary body, the eye produces less aqueous, resulting in lower intraocular pressure (IOP). Although this approach is noninvasive, the treated tissue cannot be visualized and therefore treatment titration is challenging. Treatment with TSCPC commonly results in either over treatment or under treatment, the former leading to hypotony, inflammation, and vision loss and the latter requiring further treatment. As such, TSCPC has historically been reserved for eyes with end-stage disease and limited visual potential.

ECP was designed to allow for greater control and fewer complications compared to TSCPC. The microprobe diode laser endoscopy system (EndoOptiks Inc, Little Silver, NJ) utilizes an 810-nm diode laser coupled with a 175-W xenon light source and helium neon laser-aiming beam. Using this single endoprobe, the surgeon can both visualize and treat the ciliary body. There are now 3 probe sizes that can be employed. The 19-gauge probe offers a depth of focus between 1 to 30 mm and a field of view of 110 degrees while the 20-gauge probe provides a depth of focus ranging between 0.5 to 15.0 mm and gives a field of view of 70 degrees. Recently, a 23-gauge probe has been made that is capable of inserting through all standard 23-gauge trocar systems. Straight and curved probes are available, with the latter providing greater flexibility to treat a wider angle of the ciliary processes through one incision and the ability to access a nasal wound for treating the temporal quadrant.

With the use of ECP, the surgeon is able to visualize the treated area and minimize or avoid collateral damage both within the eye and to the external conjunctiva. By targeting and treating only the visualized ciliary processes, damage to the ciliary muscle and vascular arcades can be avoided. This decreases the sometimes significant inflammatory response that can be seen with TSCPC.

In contrast to other MIGS procedures, ECP lowers IOP by decreasing aqueous production. This offers surgeons a novel approach that is effective alone or can be used to augment or potentiate other procedures aimed at increasing aqueous outflow. Similar to more recent MIGS procedures, ECP can be performed through a self-sealing clear corneal incision and easily combined with

Kahook MY.
MIGS: Advances in Glaucoma Surgery (pp 77-86).

standard cataract surgery. The added time to cataract surgery is minimal and after the initial equipment purchase has been made, all necessary instrumentation is reusable, thereby avoiding one-time costs of an implant or disposable components.

Procedure

Anesthesia

ECP has traditionally been performed with the use of a retrobulbar or sub-Tenon's block. This provides excellent intraoperative and postoperative anesthesia. If wishing to avoid the inherent risks with these injections, topical anesthesia may at times be tolerated. Adequate anesthesia can be achieved using a combination of intracameral lidocaine and brief increased sedation during the laser treatment. As the patients can have significant pain following the procedure, a mild narcotic can be prescribed following the case.

Instrumentation

- ECP instrumentation, including endoprobe, attached ECP unit, foot pedal, and monitor
- Surgical microscope
- Cohesive viscoelastic
- Sideport or keratome blade
- Irrigation and aspiration handpiece
- Balanced salt solution on an anterior chamber cannula

Setup and Settings

1. Set the laser to continuous mode and the power to 0.25 watts. This can be titrated to the observed tissue response, although the power is not commonly set higher than 0.3 to 0.35 watts.
2. The camera focus of the probe is achieved outside the eye by aiming the probe at a piece of sterile paper with printed words and rotating the focusing handle until the words come into focus.
3. The white balance can also be adjusted initially outside the eye, but this typically requires fine adjustments once the ciliary processes are in view.
4. Before insertion, the image orientation can be set using a paper with printed words to ensure proper orientation upon entering the eye. After the probe is placed in the eye, the orientation of the image is adjusted so that the ciliary processes are properly oriented in a vertical fashion. This requires constant adjustment by the surgical circulating nurse as the probe progresses around the eye. With experience, the treating surgeon will require less manipulation of camera orientation due to enhanced spatial orientation in the eye even when using a curved probe.

The Procedure

The ECP equipment is typically placed next to the phacoemulsification machine in the operating room and prepared for use prior to initiation of surgery (Figure 9-1). If combined with cataract surgery, the cataract wound can be used to treat up to 270 degrees. The arc of treatment is

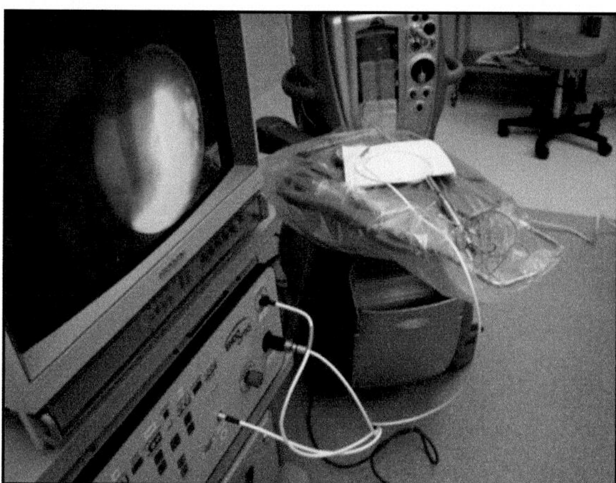

Figure 9-1. The ECP unit is positioned adjacent to the phacoemulsification unit to allow for streamlined progression from cataract to glaucoma surgery, (Reprinted with permission from Malik Y. Kahook, MD.)

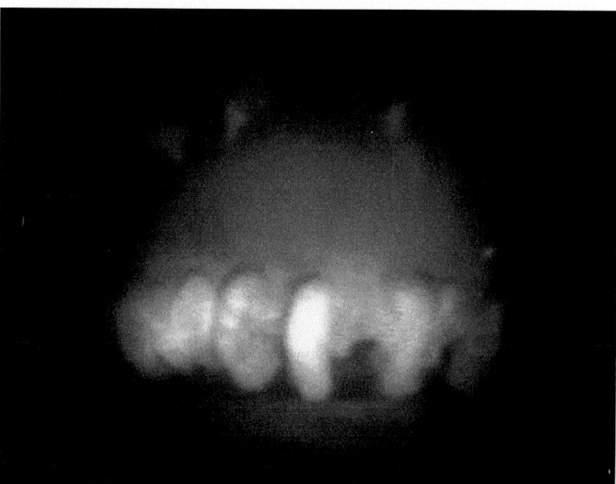

Figure 9-2. Endoscopic view of ciliary processes showing the central aiming beam with treated ciliary processes on the left and untreated processes on the right. The iris is elevated far away from the area of treatment.

larger when using the curved endoprobe compared to the straight tip. If additional treatment is desired, a supra-nasal incision can be made. The incision should be at least 1.5 mm. The cohesive viscoelastic is injected into the ciliary sulcus to deepen the space (elevating the iris away from the ciliary processes is a key step in the procedure) and improve access and visualization of the ciliary processes (Figure 9-2). The endoscope screen is positioned to ensure a good view for the surgeon. The probe is placed in the eye through the previously created incision while using the microscope. Attention is then directed toward the monitor. The probe is advanced until ~6 ciliary processes are visualized on the screen (Figures 9-3 and 9-4), indicating an approximate distance of 2 mm from the target. The processes are then treated, including the recesses in between, until they contract and whiten. Laser delivery is controlled by the foot pedal, which is held down to deliver continuous laser energy. Advancing the probe toward the processes increases the power delivered and can lead to inadvertent over treatment. Audible popping sounds and rupture of ciliary processes can occur as a result of over treatment. Treatment can be carried out in one continuous arc or split over 2 passes in opposite directions starting across from the wound. The surgical circulating nurse or assistant is needed to continuously adjust the screen orientation as the probe moves across the eye. After the treatment is concluded, the probe is withdrawn from the eye while watching through the microscope to ensure the probe is removed without any attachments to iris or lens. Finally, the viscoelastic is removed with the irrigation and aspiration handpiece. The wound can typically be closed with hydration using balanced salt solution on a 27-gauge cannula. If this fails to seal the wound, an interrupted 10-0 nylon suture is placed. Note that incomplete removal of viscoelastic is the most common cause of postoperative IOP spikes and it might be desirable, in some cases such

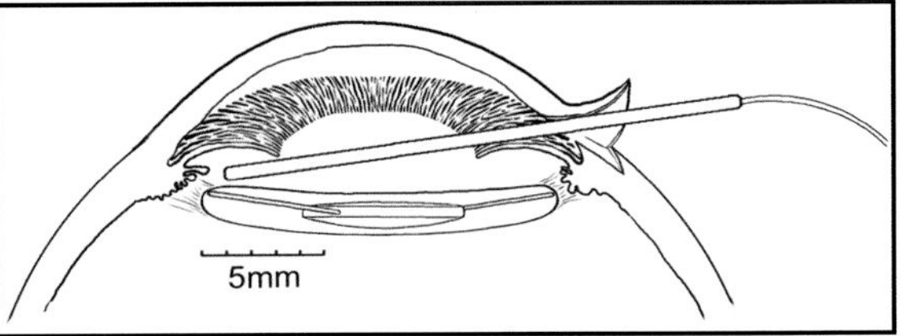

Figures 9-3. Cross-sectional view of the ECP probe in position for treatment of the ciliary processes. (Reprinted with permission from Yu JY, Kahook MY, Lathrop KL, Noecker RJ. The effect of probe placement and type of viscoelastic material on endoscopic cyclophotocoagulation laser energy transmission. *Ophthalmic Surg Lasers Imaging*. 2008;39(2):133-136.)

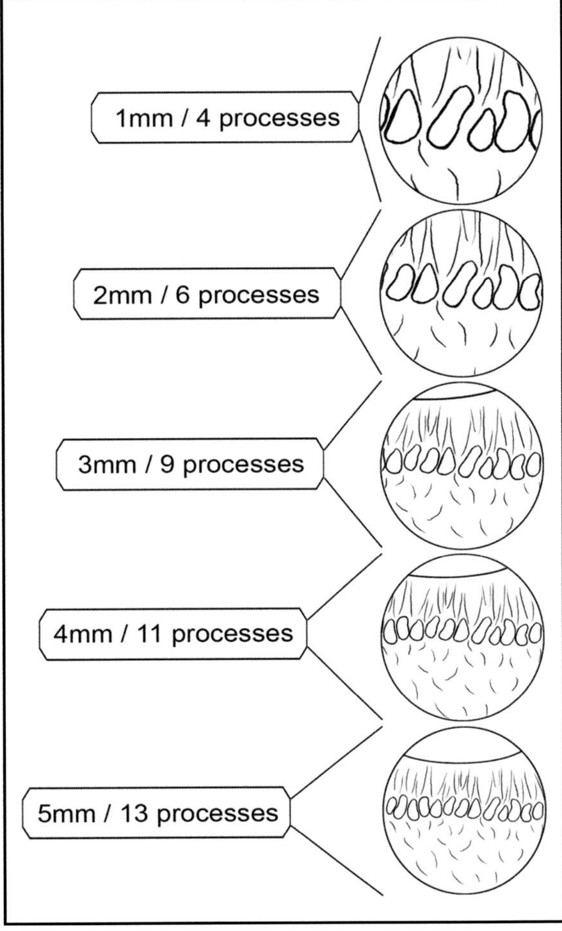

Figure 9-4. The relationship of the number of visualized ciliary processes to the distance from the probe. The appropriate treatment distance is 2 mm when 6 ciliary processes are in view. (Reprinted with permission from Yu JY, Kahook MY, Lathrop KL, Noecker RJ. The effect of probe placement and type of viscoelastic material on endoscopic cyclophotocoagulation laser energy transmission. *Ophthalmic Surg Lasers Imaging*. 2008;39(2):133-136.)

as unicameral eyes where removal of viscoelastic is difficult, to use iris hooks for elevation of the iris (Figure 9-5).

Pars Plana Approach and Endocyclophotocoagulation Plus

If more aggressive IOP lowering is required, ECP plus should be considered. This approach is especially useful in the setting of patients for whom multiple glaucoma surgeries have been unsuccessful.[1] ECP plus requires patients that are aphakic or pseudophakic. Access to the ciliary processes is gained via a pars plana approach. A sclerotomy is made 3 to 3.5 mm posterior to the limbus through the pars plana with a core anterior vitrectomy being performed. Once the vitrectomy is complete, the ECP probe is inserted via the pars plana incision. The treatment area includes the ciliary processes as well as the anterior 1 to 2 mm of pars plana, just posterior to the processes. Because this treatment is more aggressive, 360-degree treatment should be avoided in uveitic

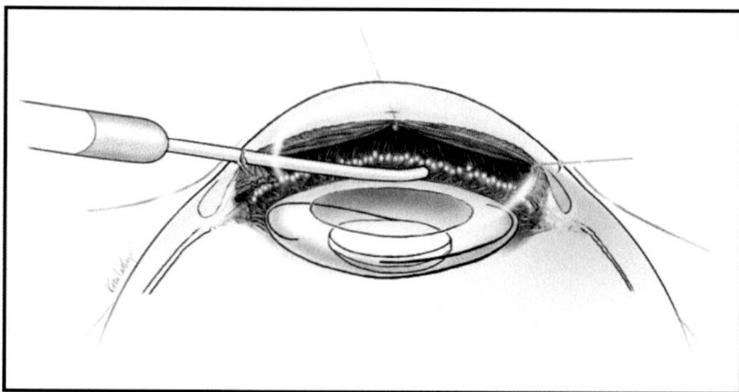

Figure 9-5. Iris hooks can be used to elevate the iris and allow for treatment of ciliary processes without or with minimal use of viscoelastic. (Reprinted with permission from Kahook MY, Schuman JS, Noecker RJ. Endoscopic cyclophotocoagulation using iris hooks versus viscoelastic devices. *Ophthalmic Surg Lasers Imaging*. 2007;38(2):170-172.)

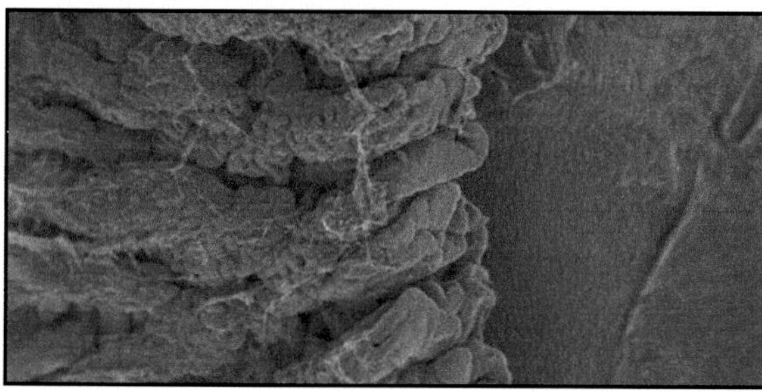

Figure 9-6. Scanning electron microscopy of ciliary processes showing blunting of the tips without collateral damage to the iris and surrounding structures. (Reprinted with permission from Malik Y. Kahook, MD.)

glaucoma. Additionally, as inflammation is typically more severe, aggressive steroid therapy may be required. This may include IV, oral, sub-Tenon's, and/or intracameral routes of administration.

Postoperative Care

Treatment postoperatively includes cycloplegia, topical antibiotics, and either frequent topical or sub-Tenon's corticosteroids. Due to occasional IOP spikes, oral acetazolamide may be given postoperatively and topical glaucoma medications may need to be continued until the IOP effect is realized. Intense steroid use can help control resulting inflammation, and these should be tapered as the inflammation resolves. The IOP-lowering effects of the procedure are typically seen between 1 to 4 weeks postoperatively.[2,3] The total effect may be blunted initially as a concomitant steroid response may also be present. Thus steroid therapy should be discontinued safely before the final effect may be realized.

Preclinical Studies

Histologic studies have shown that there is less tissue disruption in eyes treated with ECP compared to TSCPC. Looking at postmortem eyes treated at the time of autopsy, Pantcheva et al showed that the ECP-treated eyes exhibited less architectural destruction and disorganization, including sparing of the ciliary body muscle (Figures 9-6 and 9-7).[4] In a review of 9 enucleated eyes previously treated with TSCPC, McKelvie et al showed injury to the pars plicata with variable destruction of the pars plana.[5] Increasing ciliary epithelial regeneration, albeit in a disorganized pattern, was seen the further removed from the surgical date. In rabbit eyes both modalities have been shown to cause coagulation necrosis, ciliary body atrophy, and destruction to the ciliary endothelium vasculature, although more pronounced in those treated with TSCPC.[6-8] The eyes treated with ECP showed late reperfusion both by histology and endoscopic fluorescein angiography, likely explaining the more modest long-term IOP-lowering effect of ECP.

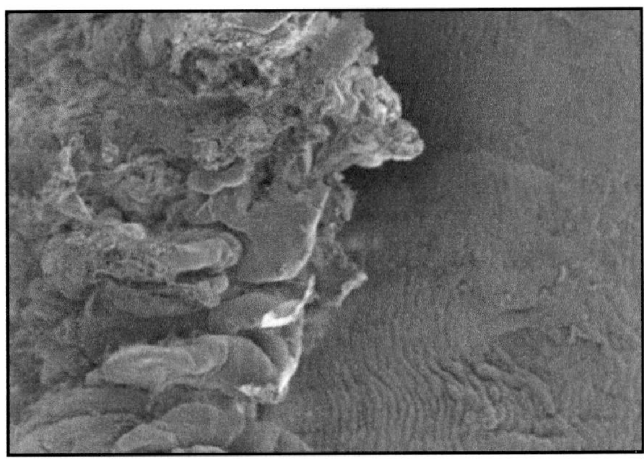

Figure 9-7. Scanning electron microscopy of ciliary processes showing widespread collateral damage with collateral damage to the iris and ciliary body. (Reprinted with permission from Malik Y. Kahook, MD.)

Clinical Studies

Retrospective Studies

There is a growing body of literature that illustrates the IOP-lowering effect of ECP seen clinically. A retrospective review of 68 eyes (12 of whom also received concurrent cataract surgery) treated with ECP showed a decrease in IOP by an average of 10.7 points for a 34% total reduction.[2] IOP-lowering medication was reduced from an average of 3 to 2 drops. Visual acuity was stable or improved in 64 eyes (94%) and decreased by greater than 2 lines in 4 patients (6%). Five eyes required a second laser procedure for IOP control. Complications included cystoid macular edema in 10%, choroidal detachment in 4%, hyphema in 12%, and fibrin exudation in 24%. There were no cases of hypotony or phthisis in this series. Although rare, Ahmad et al reported a case of phthisis 5 months after a single 360-degree ECP treatment.[9]

Kahook et al compared 2-site versus 1-site ECP in combination with phacoemulsification. Their cohort included 15 patients that received ECP through a single incision and 25 patients that received ECP through 2 incisions. At 3 months of follow-up, the group that received 2-site ECP had a lower IOP (average of 13 versus 16 mm Hg) and required less medication use (average of 0.52 versus 1.93) compared to the 1-site ECP group. They concluded that 2-site ECP with 360-degree treatment successfully reduced the IOP better than 1-site ECP.[10]

There also seems to be utility of using ECP to control IOP in patients with refractory glaucoma despite previous tube shunt placement. In these patients, Francis et al showed good results in 25 eyes receiving 360-degree ECP. Average IOP decreased from 24 to 15.4 mm Hg, representing a slightly greater than 30% reduction with an average follow-up of 12 months.[11]

Overall, these studies show that ECP is effective whether combined with cataract surgery or as an adjunct to previous filtering surgery. Additionally, 2-site ECP, with its resulting 360-degree treatment, can yield superior IOP reduction compared to 1-site ECP.

Prospective Comparative Studies

Further validating the efficacy of ECP, a few prospective studies have also shown a significant IOP reduction with this treatment. In a 2-year randomized study, Gayton et al compared ECP treatment of 240 to 270 degrees of ciliary processes to trabeculectomy in 58 eyes. Both were performed at the time of cataract surgery.[12] The success rate in lowering IOP to less than 19 mm Hg without medications was 42% in the trabeculectomy group compared to 30% in the ECP group. The same level of IOP control with medications was achieved in 65% of the ECP group compared to 54% in the trabeculectomy group. Treatment failure occurred in 14% of ECP patients and 10% of trabeculectomy patients who required additional surgical intervention.

Another prospective study compared ECP to Ahmed valve (New World Medical, Inc, Rancho Cucamonga, CA) placement in patients who had received previous trabeculectomy.[3] The authors included 68 eyes in 68 patients with refractory glaucoma, a pressure of at least 35 mm Hg on maximal medical therapy, and vision of light perception or better. Preoperative IOP was an average of 41 mm Hg in both groups. Patients with a previous drainage implant or cyclodestructive procedure were excluded from the study. Success was defined as an IOP between 6 and 21 mm Hg with or without medications. Average IOP at 2 years in the Ahmed group was 14.7 and 14.1 mm Hg in the ECP group. The Kaplan-Meier survival curves predicted a success rate of 70.6% in the Ahmed group and 73.5% in the ECP group at 2 years. The Ahmed group had a higher risk of choroidal detachment (17.6% versus 2.9%) but lower risk of hyphema (14.7% versus 17.6%).

This limited but significant evidence suggests that ECP can achieve IOP control comparable to traditional filtering procedures, although medications are often still required to attain target IOP in the ECP-treated groups.

Alternative Uses of the Endocyclophotocoagulation Probe

In addition to its predominant role in cyclophotocoagulation, the ECP probe can be utilized to diagnose and treat a variety of ocular conditions. It is particularly helpful in exploring the ciliary sulcus and in other conditions where visibility is otherwise limited. As a therapeutic modality, it is useful in the setting of uveitis-glaucoma-hyphema (UGH) syndrome, small cyclodialysis clefts, and plateau iris among other things.

Ciliary Sulcus and Anterior Segment Procedures

By virtue of its location behind the iris, the ciliary sulcus can be difficult, if not impossible, to visualize without the capabilities of the endoscope. Using the ECP probe, surgeons can very easily explore this vital area of the eye. This is particularly useful in UGH syndrome, a condition often caused by iris chafing from sulcus-placed intraocular lenses (IOLs) abutting the iris. In several cases at our institution, by using the endoscope possible cases of UGH syndrome were effectively confirmed upon localization of the offending haptics. Additionally, under visualization with the endoscope, microincisional forceps and scissors were used to successfully remove the haptics and the condition halted.

Sulcus-placed IOLs are traditionally placed when the integrity of the posterior capsule is compromised. Although these lenses occasionally lead to UGH syndrome, 3-piece sulcus IOLs typically do well. Sometimes, however, it is challenging to determine if the sulcus shelf, including the anterior capsule and the lens zonules, is able to support a sulcus IOL without risking future dislocation. Once again, the ECP probe is ideal for this setting. Using the probe, the stability and integrity of the sulcus can be visualized and assessed prior to the insertion of a 3-piece IOL.

The ECP probe has proven useful in another rare but important use. In a case at one of our centers, a patient was struck in the eye by a small metallic foreign body. It penetrated his cornea, leading to a self-sealing wound. Unknown at the time, the fragment then penetrated the iris and came to rest in the ciliary sulcus, near the zonules. The patient's eye was quiet for a number of months until it started to develop signs of early siderosis. The decision was then made to retrieve the foreign body. The endoprobe successfully localized the foreign body and the piece was successfully retrieved with the use of an intraocular magnet.

Another novel use of the ECP probe is in the diagnosis and treatment of epithelial downgrowth. This has been previously reported in the literature in a case with a dense corneal opacity.[13] In a similar case at our institution, we successfully used ECP to treat epithelial downgrowth associated with a recent penetrating keratoplasty. The patient presented with a membrane over the inferior corneal endothelium, which quickly involved the central cornea. The ECP handpiece was used to apply continuous laser to the involved structures, including the corneal endothelium, iris face, and angle. Diagnostic whitening of the affected membrane was noted during the procedure, after which this membrane was removed. Additional treatment was applied to the involved areas along the posterior surface of the iris. Following this, a new penetrating keratoplasty was performed. There were no signs of recurrence after 1 year.

The ECP probe is also useful for closing small cyclodialysis clefts. It has been previously reported to aid in direct visualization and treatment of a cyclodialysis cleft measuring 2.5 clock hours.[14] The ECP probe was crucial in one such closure at our center. An 8-year-old boy presented with traumatic cleft. His IOP was 3 mm Hg accompanied by retinal striae, optic nerve edema, and decreased visual acuity to 20/125. The ECP probe successfully identified a cleft of a single clock hour. Using standard settings (power 0.2 to 0.4 watts on continuous mode), laser was applied to the area of the cyclodialysis cleft, resulting in shrinkage of the peripheral iris. After an initial postoperative pressure spike, indicating closure of the cleft, the patient stabilized with an IOP of 16 mm Hg on timolol and a visual acuity of 20/25.

It is apparent that the ECP probe is useful in a variety of anterior segment scenarios. Cases of epithelial downgrowth, UGH syndrome, sulcus investigation, cyclodialysis cleft closure, as well as many other uses are facilitated and in many cases made possible with the use of the endoscopic probe.

Pediatric Use

Refractory pediatric glaucoma is an ideal setting for the use of ECP. In a retrospective analysis, Carter et al helped validate the role of ECP in a pediatric population with aphakic and pseudophakic glaucoma. The study included 34 eyes in 25 patients under age 16, with a goal IOP < 24 mm Hg. They showed an overall success rate of 38% in patients receiving only one treatment and up to 53% in eyes receiving repeat treatment. IOP declined from an average of 32.6 to 22.9 mm Hg at an average follow-up of 44 months. There were no cases of hypotony; however, retinal detachments developed in 2 eyes.[15]

Other studies of pediatric glaucoma have confirmed similar reductions in IOP. It has been reported to be particularly useful in eyes with corneal opacities, such as Peter's anomaly and other anterior segment dysgenesis. The ECP probe has been used both in treating the ciliary body in a traditional fashion and by using the endoscopic camera to assist in the placement of anterior chamber tube shunts.[16]

Retinal Use

Retinal surgeons rely heavily on the clarity of the cornea to visualize and treat retinal pathology. When the cornea is compromised, it can be difficult to safely perform pars plana vitrectomy. The endoscope has successfully been employed in such conditions to allow the surgeon the ability to image, illuminate, and apply laser treatment to the retina. Retinal surgeons have successfully used the endoscope to explore and treat retinal detachments and endophthalmitis and assist in vitrectomy prior to pars plana insertion of tube shunts in cases with opaque corneas. These types of cases would otherwise be difficult if not impossible to perform.[17-19]

Plateau Iris

Plateau iris is a condition in which anterior or large ciliary processes cause anterior rotation of the peripheral iris. It is a cause of angle closure that traditionally does not respond to a peripheral iridotomy alone. Ultrasound biomicroscopy has shown that cataract surgery alone is not curative in these cases.[20]

Cataract surgery combined with ECP can help alleviate this condition by shrinking these anteriorly displaced processes. Using the ECP probe in this condition is referred to as endocycloplasty (ECPL). In this procedure the laser energy is applied to the posterior portion of the ciliary processes until the anterior portion of the processes shrink and rotate posteriorly. The goal is to shrink the processes without causing the destruction of traditional ECP. This pulls the entire process posteriorly away from the iris, restoring appropriate angle anatomy. A retrospective review of ECPL in 58 eyes with 3 months of follow-up showed improvement in IOP (17.3 to 13.3 mm Hg). Complications were mild and self-limiting. The angle widened considerably by gonioscopy, improving from a Schaffer classification of 0.92 to 2.82. Although these results are early and retrospective in nature, the results are promising.[21]

Additionally, given the success of this procedure in widening the angle, conceivably, once the angle anatomy is restored, ab interno canal-based surgery could be considered.

Comparison to Other Ab Interno Procedures

As with other ab interno surgical procedures, ECP through a clear cornea approach avoids damage to the conjunctiva that may be necessary for future ab externo glaucoma procedures. Equally, it spares the trabecular meshwork and Schlemm's canal that could be used for either ab externo (eg, canaloplasty) or ab interno canal-based surgery (eg, iStent [Glaukos Corp, Laguna Hills, CA] or Trabectome [NeoMedix Corp, Tustin, CA]). As ECP can be easily combined with cataract surgery, adding little additional time or incisions, it is a simple procedure that can provide significant benefit to patients with concomitant cataracts and mild-to-moderate glaucoma. It can likewise be used in refractory glaucoma patients for whom further scleral-based surgery is not possible or undesired.

Although the initial body of clinical evidence for the safety and efficacy of ECP is promising, future studies are needed. More prospective trials with longer follow-up will help to better define the patient populations ideal for this treatment. Randomized and controlled studies can further isolate the IOP-lowering effect of ECP from cataract surgery alone. Nevertheless, the ECP probe is a valuable tool for any ophthalmic surgeon and a unique addition to the MIGS arsenal.

References

1. Spaeth G, Uram M. Use of endocyclophotocoagulation in patients with uncontrolled refractory glaucoma. Poster presented at: American Glaucoma Society 16th Annual Meeting; March 4, 2006; Charleston, SC.
2. Chen J, Cohn RA, Lin SC, Cortes AE, Alvarado JA. Endoscopic photocoagulation of the ciliary body for treatment of refractory glaucomas. *Am J Ophthalmol.* 1997;124:787–796.
3. Lima FE, Magacho L, Carvalho DM, Susanna R, Jr, Avila MP. A prospective, comparative study between endoscopic cyclophotocoagulation and the Ahmed drainage implant in refractory glaucoma. *J Glaucoma.* 2004;13:233–237.
4. Pantcheva MB, Kahook MK, Schuman JS, Noecker RJ. Comparison of acute structural and histopathological changes in human autopsy eyes after endoscopic cyclophotocoagulation and trans-scleral cyclophotocoagulation. *Br J Ophthalmol.* 2007;91:248–252.
5. McKelvie PA, Walland MJ. Pathology of cyclodiode laser: a series of nine enucleated eyes. *Br J Ophthalmol.* 2002;86(4):381-86.

6. Schlote T, Beck J, Rohrbach JM, Funk RH. Alteration of the vascular supply in the rabbit ciliary body by transscleral diode laser cyclophotocoagulation. *Graefes Arch Clin Exp Ophthalmol.* 2001;239(1):53-58.
7. Lin SC, Chen MJ, Lin MS, Howes E, Stamper RL. Vascular effects of ciliary tissue from endoscopic versus transscleral cyclophotocoagulation. *Br J Opthalmol.* 2006;90:496–500.
8. Schuman JS, Jacobson JJ, Puliafito CA, Noecker RJ, Reidy WT. Experimental use of semiconductor diode laser in contact transscleral cyclophotocoagulation in rabbits. *Arch Ophthalmol.* 1990;108(8):1152-1157.
9. Ahmad S, Wallace DJ, Herndon LW. Phthisis after endoscopic cyclophotocoagulation. *Ophthalmic Surg Lasers Imaging.* 2008;39:407-408.
10. Kahook MY, Lathrop KL, Noecker RJ. One-site versus two-site endoscopic cyclophotocoagulation. *J Glaucoma.* 2007;16:527–530.
11. Francis BA, Kawji AS, Vo NT, Dustin L, Chopra V. Endoscopic cyclophotocoagulation (ECP) in the management of uncontrolled glaucoma with prior aqueous tube shunt. *J Glaucoma.* 2011; 20:523-527.
12. Gayton JL, Van De Karr M, Sanders V. Combined cataract and glaucoma surgery: trabeculectomy versus endoscopic laser cycloablation. *J Cataract Refract Surg.* 1999;25:1214–1219.
13. Jadav DS, Rylander NR, Vold SD, Fulcher SF, Rosa RH Jr. Endoscopic photocoagulation in the management of epithelial downgrowth. *Cornea.* 2008;27:601-604.
14. Caronia RM, Sturm RT, Marmor MA, Berke SJ. Treatment of a cyclodialysis cleft by means of ophthalmic laser microendoscope endophotocoagulation. *Am J Ophthalmol.* 1999;128:760-761.
15. Carter BC, Plager DA, Neely DE, Sprunger DT, Sondhi N, Roberts GJ. Endoscopic diode laser cyclophotocoagulation in the management of aphakic and pseudophakic glaucoma in children. *J AAPOS.* 2007;11:34-40
16. Al-Haddad CE, Freedman SF. Endoscopic laser cyclophotocoagulation in pediatric glaucoma with corneal opacities. *J AAPOS.* 2007;11:23-28.
17. Kita M, Yoshimura N. Endoscope-assisted vitrectomy in the management of pseudophakic and aphakic retinal detachments with undetected retinal breaks. *Retina.* 2011;31:1347-1351.
18. Tarantola RM, Agarwal A, Lu P, Joos KM. Long-term results of combined endoscope-assisted pars plana vitrectomy and glaucoma tube shunt surgery. *Retina.* 2011;31:275-283.
19. De Smet MD, Carlborg EA. Managing severe endophthalmitis with the use of an endoscope. *Retina.* 2005;25:976-980.
20. Tran HV, Liebmann JM, Ritch R. Iridociliary apposition in plateau iris syndrome persists after cataract extraction. *Am J Ophthalmol.* 2003;135(1):40-43.
21. Ahmed IIK, Podbielski DW, Naqi A, et al. Endoscopic cycloplasty in angle closure glaucoma secondary to plateau iris. Poster presented at: AGS Annual Meeting; March 5-8, 2009; San Diego, CA.

10

Cataract Surgery as a MIGS Procedure

John P. Berdahl, MD

Cataracts are the most common surgical procedure in the United States, while glaucoma affects nearly 2% of the population over age 65.[1,2] Therefore, it is not surprising that these conditions are often present simultaneously. Cataracts are the leading cause of blindness worldwide, while glaucoma is the second leading cause of blindness worldwide, with glaucoma being the number one cause of irreversible blindness. Surgeons commonly encounter patients with early cataracts and progressive glaucoma and become tasked with identifying the best next step. Studies have shown that cataract surgery alone can lower intraocular pressure (IOP), and the most recent data indicate that IOP reduction after cataract surgery may be more sustained than previously recognized.[3-6]

The goal of glaucoma therapy has been to prevent visual field loss by lowering IOP. Trabeculectomy and tube shunts have been the typical method of lowering IOP surgically; however, these procedures carry significant risk. The 5-year results of the tube versus trabeculectomy trial have shown that 47% of trabeculectomies and 30% of tube shunts fail at 5 years.[7] More recently, MIGS such as the iStent (Glaukos Corporation, Laguna Hills, CA) and Trabectome (NeoMedix Corporation, Tustin, CA), have become available and may lead to a safer way to lower IOP than traditional surgical approaches.[4]

Our understanding of the relationship between cataracts and glaucoma has evolved over time. Because many patients with cataracts also have glaucoma, some have suggested that glaucoma itself is a risk factor for progression of cataracts, although mechanisms are unclear.[8] A more likely explanation is that cataract and glaucoma occur in patients with similar demographics and because glaucoma patients receive more regular exams, an early cataract is less likely to be missed. Cataract development is known to increase following filtering procedures and peripheral iridotomies, possibly as a result of aqueous diversion through peripheral iridotomy, resulting in decreased metabolic functions of the anterior lens or other factors such as inflammation or topical steroid use.[9-11]

Traditional options for patients with concurrent cataract and progressive glaucoma have been either a combined cataract and trabeculectomy (or tube shunt) or a staged procedure.[12,13] Neither combined cataract and glaucoma surgery or staged procedures have demonstrated a clear superiority over one another. Given the tepid results from the tube versus trabeculectomy trial,[7] many surgeons are eager to avoid tubes or trabeculectomies whenever possible. However, because the

Kahook MY.
MIGS: Advances in Glaucoma Surgery (pp 87-91).

dogma has been that cataract surgery alone lowers IOP temporarily and only slightly, phacoemulsification alone was not considered a good option to treat glaucoma.[14]

Recent data show a greater and more sustained IOP reduction following cataract surgery alone than previously thought.[3,4,15] Therefore, cataract surgery alone may be preferable to a combined cataract surgery with tube shunt or trabeculectomy and may be the original minimally invasive glaucoma surgery.

Early studies of the IOP response to cataract surgery showed little reduction to IOP.[16-18] These early data were obtained in the era of large-incision extracapsular cataract surgery and probably do not apply to today's more controlled microincisional phacoemulsification. (Interestingly, we may be entering an era where traditional phacoemulsification data may not apply with the advent of femtosecond-assisted cataract extraction.) As extracapsular cataract surgery became more commonly used, studies started to demonstrate decreased IOP of 2 to 3 mm Hg for about 2 years.[19] There has been one meta-analysis of this topic that confirmed the traditional teaching. The meta-analysis itself had significant limitations, including that long-term was defined as over 24 hours (although many studies had longer follow-up), which probably has little bearing on glaucoma progression.[14] The data in the meta-analysis also only interpreted mean values, and patients were not stratified based on preoperative IOP. When data were stratified based on preoperative IOP, those patients with the highest preoperative IOP had the greatest IOP reduction from cataract surgery. Longer-term studies showed a drop of nearly 3 mm Hg in glaucoma patients.[3,20,21] The method of cataract extraction may influence how IOP responds. Clear-cornea phacoemulsification appears to lower IOP more than manual extracapsular cataract extraction. No data are available on femtosecond techniques for cataract extraction yet. Additionally, the type of glaucoma may affect IOP reduction. Pseudoexfoliation patients may have an even larger decrease in IOP than other types of glaucoma patients, despite the tendency to have an IOP spike in the perioperative period.[22,23] Anecdotally, hyperopes that have a smaller anterior chamber may also disproportionately benefit from cataract surgery as a means to lower IOP.

The largest and most recent studies have demonstrated sustained IOP lowering[3,6] with some exceptions.[24] In a large retrospective study, Poley et al[3] showed that stratifying patients by preoperative IOP demonstrated a larger drop in IOP from phacoemulsification when preoperative IOP was higher (Table 10-1). This was confirmed in an analysis of the Ocular Hypertensive Treatment Trial data, which showed that in the cataract group, postoperative IOP was significantly lower than the preoperative IOP (19.8 ± 3.2 mm Hg versus 23.9 ± 3.2 mm Hg; $P < 0.001$). The postoperative IOP remained lower than the preoperative IOP for at least 36 months, and those with the highest preoperative IOP showed the greatest reduction following phacoemulsification.[6]

Removal of a cataract (and in some cases a clear lens) in the setting of chronic and acute angle-closure glaucoma has been shown to decrease IOP and prevent future episodes of angle closure. One recent study showed that both phacoemulsification and trabeculectomy are effective in reducing IOP in medically uncontrolled chronic angle-closure glaucoma eyes.[25] Trabeculectomy is more effective than phacoemulsification in reducing dependence on glaucoma drugs, but is associated with more complications.[25] Another study showed that cataract surgery performed within 1 week of acute angle closure, coexisting cataract, phaco/IOL surgery resulted in a lower rate of IOP failure at 2 years compared with laser peripheral iridotomy.[26]

The exact physiologic reason for decreased IOP following cataract surgery has not been clearly elucidated. Three possible mechanisms that could contribute to reduced IOP after cataract surgery are listed next.

Table 10-1.

INTRAOCULAR PRESSURE DECREASE AFTER PHACOEMULSIFICATION STRATIFIED BY PREOPERATIVE INTRAOCULAR PRESSURE

		MEAN ± SD						
				IOP (mm Hg)				
IOP (mm Hg) Group	*Eyes (n)*	*Age (Y)*	*Postop FU (Y)*	*At Surgery*	*1 Y Postop*	*Change at 1 Y*	*Final*	*Change Final (%)*
31 to 23	19	69.3 ± 7.4	2.4 ± 2.4	24.5 ± 2.1	17.8 ± 3.2	-6.7 ± 3.1	18.0 ± 2.8	-6.5 ± 2.8 (27)
22 to 20	62	70.9 ± 10.3	4.6 ± 2.2	20.9 ± 0.8	15.8 ± 3.0	-5.1 ± 2.9	16.1 ± 2.7	-4.8 ± 2.5 (22)
19 to 18	86	67.4 ± 11.6	4.9 ± 2.9	18.3 ± 0.4	15.5 ± 2.3	-2.8 ± 2.3	15.8 ± 2.4	-2.5 ± 2.5 (14)
17 to 15	223	71.2 ± 9.9	4.7 ± 2.6	15.9 ± 0.7	14.6 ± 2.4	-1.4 ± 2.4	14.3 ± 2.6	-1.6 ± 2.6 (10)
14 to 9	198	70.5 ± 10.5	4.2 ± 2.6	12.7 ± 1.4	13.1 ± 2.6	+0.4 ± 2.6	12.9 ± 2.5	+0.2 ± 2.6 (0)
P value	—	.57	.002	< .001	< .001	< .001	< .001	< .001
All eyes	588	70.3 ± 10.4	4.5 ± 2.6	16.0 ± 3.1	14.5 ± 2.8	-1.5 ± 3.2	14.4 ± 2.9	-1.6 ± 3.1 (10)

FU = follow-up; IOP = intraocular pressure

Reprinted with permission from Poley BJ, Lindstrom RL, Samuelson TW. Long-term effects of phacoemulsification with intraocular lens implantation in normotensive and ocular hypertensive eyes. *J Cataract Refract Surg.* 2008;34:735–742.

Lens-Induced Changes to the Outflow Pathway

With age, the crystalline lens becomes thicker and increases significantly in volume (Figure 10-1). The anatomical changes that accompany the increase in size of the lens may lead to a direct congestion of the outflow pathway.[27] The increasing anterior/posterior diameter may cause the accompanying anterior zonules to create anteriorly directed traction on the ciliary body and uvea, which could compress Schlemm's canal and possibly the trabecular meshwork.[28] Anatomically, this is logical because the anterior tendons of the ciliary muscle contribute to the trabecular meshwork architecture. Hence, as the ciliary body moves forward from the enlarged lens, the tendons can relax and the spaces between trabecular plates can become narrowed.

Cataract Surgery-Induced Inflammation

Phacoemulsification typically induces a low-grade inflammation immediately postoperatively. It is possible that it is this induced inflammation that may lower IOP by either decreasing aqueous production from the ciliary body (similar to uveitis), or it could increase outflow similar to the mechanism of selective laser trabeculoplasty and prostaglandin analogs.

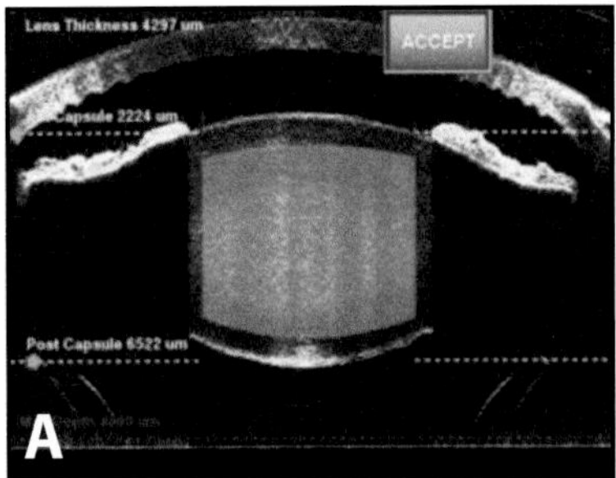
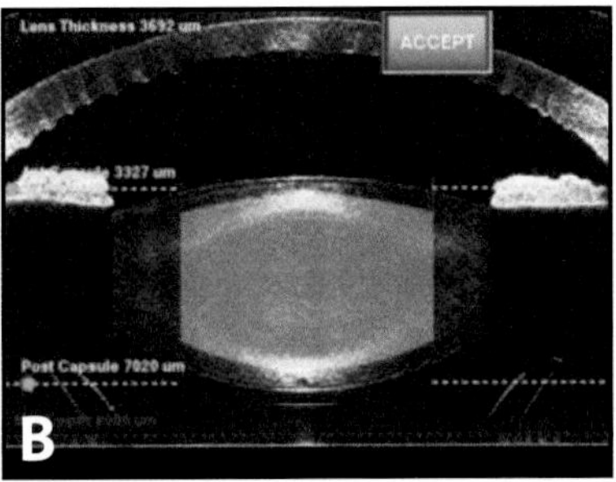

Figure 10-1. Anterior segment optical coherence tomography of a (A) 90 year old and (B) a 60 year old showing marked differences in lens thickness.

High Flow Phacoemulsification

Another possible explanation is that high flow and high IOP (up to 80 to 90 mm Hg) during cataract surgery forces fluid through the trabecular meshwork into Schlemm's canal and through the episcleral veins. This high-pressure situation, in combination with high flow throughout the drainage system, may contribute to increased patency and increase the facility of outflow. Again, there is little experimental evidence to demonstrate this. The high flow of fluid in the anterior chamber might also lead to sheer stress on the trabecular meshwork, which subsequently leads to an increase in specific cytokines like E-Selectin.[29] Induction of specific cytokines could lead to remodeling of the extracellular matrix in the outflow pathway and subsequently decrease IOP. This has been shown to occur in preclinical testing and requires further validation in clinical studies.

Is Cataract Surgery a MIGS Procedure?

The consensus of the data is that cataract surgery lowers IOP in a significant and sustained way. Cataract surgery may be the most minimally invasive intraocular glaucoma surgery available. Although combining cataract surgery with other minimally invasive glaucoma surgeries will lead to a greater IOP reduction, in some cases cataract surgery alone may achieve the surgeon's and patient's goal of slowing progression or decreasing medications.

References

1. Quigley HA. Number of people with glaucoma worldwide. *Br J Ophthalmol.* 1996;80:389–393.
2. West S. Epidemiology of cataract: accomplishments over 25 years and future directions. *Ophthalmic Epidemiol.* 2007;14:173–178.
3. Poley BJ, Lindstrom RL, Samuelson TW. Long-term effects of phacoemulsification with intraocular lens implantation in normotensive and ocular hypertensive eyes. *J Cataract Refract Surg.* 2008;34:735–742.
4. Samuelson TW, Katz LJ, Wells JM, et al. Randomized evaluation of the trabecular micro-bypass stent with phacoemulsification in patients with glaucoma and cataract. *Ophthalmology.* 2011;118:459–467.
5. Shrivastava A, Singh K. The effect of cataract extraction on intraocular pressure. *Curr Opin Ophthalmol.* 2010;21:118–122.
6. Mansberger SL, Gordon MO, Jampel H, et al. Reduction in intraocular pressure after cataract extraction: the ocular hypertension treatment study. *Ophthalmology.* 2012;119:1826–1831.
7. Gedde SJ, Schiffman JC, Feuer WJ, et al. Treatment outcomes in the Tube Versus Trabeculectomy (TVT) study after five years of follow-up. *Am J Ophthalmol.* 2012;153:789–803.e2.
8. Hodge WG, Whitcher JP, Satariano W. Risk factors for age-related cataracts. *Epidemiol Rev.* 1995;17:336–346.

9. Jampel H. Trabeculectomy: more effective at causing cataract surgery than lowering intraocular pressure? *Ophthalmology.* 2009;116:173–174.
10. Lim LS, Husain R, Gazzard G, et al. Cataract progression after prophylactic laser peripheral iridotomy: potential implications for the prevention of glaucoma blindness. *Ophthalmology.* 2005;112:1355–1359.
11. Leske MC, Wu S-Y, Nemesure B, Hennis A. Risk factors for incident nuclear opacities. *Ophthalmology.* 2002;109:1303–1308.
12. Rosdahl JA, Chen TC. Combined cataract and glaucoma surgeries: traditional and new combinations. *Int Ophthalmol Clin.* 2010;50:95–106.
13. Wedrich A, Menapace R, Radax U, Papapanos P. Long-term results of combined trabeculectomy and small incision cataract surgery. *J Cataract Refract Surg.* 1995;21:49–54.
14. Friedman DS, Jampel HD, Lubomski LH, et al. Surgical strategies for coexisting glaucoma and cataract: an evidence-based update. *Ophthalmology.* 2002;109:1902–1913.
15. Hansen MH, Gyldenkerne GJ, Otland NW, et al. Intraocular pressure seven years after extracapsular cataract extraction and sulcus implantation of a posterior chamber intraocular lens. *J Cataract Refract Surg.* 1995;21:676–678.
16. Radius RL, Schultz K, Sobocinski K, et al. Pseudophakia and intraocular pressure. *Am J Ophthalmol.* 1984;97:738–742.
17. Bigger JF, Becker B. Cataracts and primary open-angle glaucoma: the effect of uncomplicated cataract extraction on glaucoma control. *Trans Am Acad Ophthalmol Otolaryngol.* 1971;75:260–272.
18. Randolph ME, Maumenee AE, Iliff CE. Cataract extraction in glaucomatous eyes. *Ophthalmology.* 1971;71:328–330.
19. Tennen DG, Masket S. Short-and long-term effect of clear corneal incisions on intraocular pressure. *J Cataract Refract Surg.* 1996;22:568–570.
20. Leelachaikul Y, Euswas A. Long-term intraocular pressure change after clear corneal phacoemulsification in Thai glaucoma patients. *J Med Assoc Thai.* 2005;88 Suppl 9:S21–S25.
21. Bowling B, Calladine D. Routine reduction of glaucoma medication following phacoemulsification. *J Cataract Refract Surg.* 2009;35:406–407.
22. Merkur A, Damji KF, Mintsioulis G, Hodge WG. Intraocular pressure decrease after phacoemulsification in patients with pseudoexfoliation syndrome. *J Cataract Refract Surg.* 2001;27:528–532.
23. Shingleton BJ, Heltzer J, O'Donoghue MW. Outcomes of phacoemulsification in patients with and without pseudoexfoliation syndrome. *J Cataract Refract Surg.* 2003;29:1080–1086.
24. Chang TC, Budenz DL, Liu A, et al. Long-term effect of phacoemulsification on intraocular pressure using phakic fellow eye as control. *J Cataract Refract Surg.* 2012;38:866–870.
25. Tham CCY, Kwong YYY, Baig N, et al. Phacoemulsification versus trabeculectomy in medically uncontrolled chronic angle-closure glaucoma without cataract. *Ophthalmology.* 2012.
26. Husain R, Gazzard G, Aung T, et al. Initial management of acute primary angle closure: a randomized trial comparing phacoemulsification with laser peripheral iridotomy. *Ophthalmology.* 2012;119:2274–2281.
27. Huang G, Gonzalez E, Peng P-H, et al. Anterior chamber depth, iridocorneal angle width, and intraocular pressure changes after phacoemulsification: narrow vs open iridocorneal angles. *Arch Ophthalmol.* 2011;129:1283–1290.
28. Strenk SA, Strenk LM, Guo S. Magnetic resonance imaging of the anteroposterior position and thickness of the aging, accommodating, phakic, and pseudophakic ciliary muscle. *J Cataract Refract Surg.* 2010;36:235–241.
29. Wang N, Chintala SK, Fini ME, Schuman JS. Ultrasound activates the TM ELAM-1/IL-1/NF-kappaB response: a potential mechanism for intraocular pressure reduction after phacoemulsification. *Invest Ophthalmol Vis Sci.* 2003;44(5):1977-81.

11

Emerging Surgical Interventions

Leonard K. Seibold, MD

The recent surge in development of MIGS procedures has produced many innovative devices and techniques to provide for a safer and more effective glaucoma treatment. The most well studied and established of these procedures have been described in this text in more detail. However, many other procedures have the potential to become widely used as further evaluations are performed. This chapter will introduce these novel devices and procedures and illustrate their unique features and potential for success. It should be noted that many of these are still in the infancy of their development and clinical evidence may be limited or absent. Continued efforts by their developers and the ophthalmologic community will better characterize these procedures and determine their ultimate value in the treatment of glaucoma.

Sclerothalamotomy Ab Interno

The sclerothalamotomy ab interno (STT ab interno) procedure is a modification on earlier nonpenetrating surgeries such as deep sclerectomy.[1] While the removal of perilimbal sclera is not a new concept, the ab interno approach of this procedure is what makes it unique. The aim of the procedure is to create large cavities or "thalami" through the trabecular meshwork (TM) and into the deep sclera. The scleral pocket allows aqueous to bypass any flow limitation at the TM and egress directly into exposed ends of Schlemm's canal. It is hypothesized that fluid may also drain through the ciliary body or the exposed scleral layers, which are thinned by the treatment. Advantages of STT ab interno include the relatively quick learning curve and short procedure time. The intraocular pressure (IOP)-lowering effect also has the potential to be titrated by the number of thalami created. In addition, the conjunctiva is spared, making subsequent filtering surgeries still possible.

The STT is accomplished by the use of a high frequency, intraocular diathermy probe (Oertli Instruments, Berneck, Switzerland). The probe has a 1-mm long platinum tip that is only 0.3 mm in diameter. The inner platinum electrode is isolated from the returning coaxial electrodes. A bipolar energy source then delivers a 500-kHz bipolar current to heat the probe tip to 130°C while leaving the remainder of the probe cool. The device is then inserted through at least a 1.2-mm clear corneal wound and advanced to the opposite anterior chamber angle. Intraoperative gonioscopy

Kahook MY.
MIGS: Advances in Glaucoma Surgery (pp 93-100).

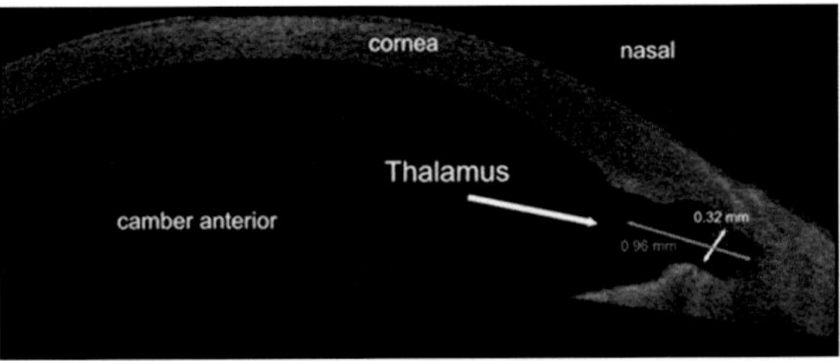

Figure 11-1. Anterior segment optical coherence tomography image of the nasal anterior chamber 6 weeks after STT ab interno. The cavity or thalamus is seen at the iridocorneal angle and measures 0.32-mm high and 0.96-mm deep.

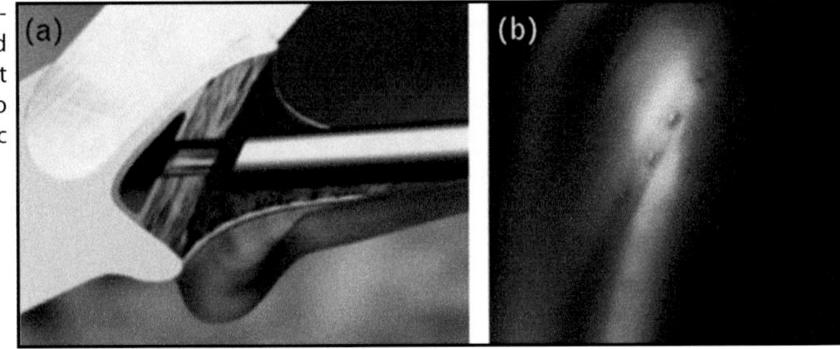

Figure 11-2. Excimer laser trabeculotomy (ELT). (A) The beveled tip of the probe is positioned next to the TM to create an opening to Schlemm's canal. (B) Gonioscopic view of TM openings from ELT.

is used to visualize the angle, and then the probe tip is advanced into the sclera and heated to create 4 sclerotomies measuring 0.3-mm deep and 0.6-mm wide. Anterior segment optical coherence tomography nicely illustrates the thalami created by this procedure (Figure 11-1).[1] Histologic analysis has not shown coagulative damage or cellular necrosis from the diathermy.[2]

Initial evidence of the clinical efficacy and safety of STT ab interno was demonstrated by Pajic et al in 2011.[1] In this study, a total of 58 eyes with either open-angle or juvenile glaucoma were treated with STT ab interno and followed for a minimum of 6 years. After 4 thalami were created, preoperative mean IOP was significantly decreased in both groups at the end of follow-up (25.6 to 14.7 mm Hg for the open-angle group and 39.6 to 13.2 mm Hg for the juvenile group). Mean number of medications fell from 2.6 preoperatively to 0.5 postoperatively at 72-month follow-up. Over 98% of treated eyes achieved an IOP level of < 21 mm Hg with medications and 79.2% of treated eyes achieve this IOP without medications. Early postoperative complications were infrequent and minor, including hyphema (11.4%) and temporary IOP elevation (22.6%). Cataract formation was the only noted late complication in 17.1% of patients, with one-third not affecting visual acuity. No serious adverse events were reported. The initially favorable efficacy and safety outcomes of this procedure will need further validation in the future.

Excimer Laser Trabeculotomy

Another ab interno MIGS procedure aimed at bypassing TM is excimer laser trabeculotomy (ELT). Despite its comparisons to selective laser trabeculoplasty (SLT), ELT is a wholly different procedure. The goal of the procedure is to create multiple 0.5-mm full-thickness holes through the TM allowing direct access for aqueous to enter Schlemm's canal and exit through downstream collector channels. The energy is delivered through a fiber optic probe connected to a xenon chloride (XeCl) excimer laser (AIDA, Glautec AG, Nurnberg, Germany). This is a pulsed laser with duration of 80 ns and an emission wavelength of 308 nm, delivering an average energy of 1.2 mJ per pulse.[3] The quartz probe is mounted in a stainless-steel casing with a beveled tip to aid in placement within the angle (Figure 11-2). The ratio of trabecular tissue to water is quite small, allowing for a cooling effect at the boundaries of the ablation zone. Thus, tissue ablation in ELT is uniquely accomplished without collateral thermal damage.

Some theoretical advantages of ELT are its internal approach, the ablation of TM without thermal damage, short procedure time, and potential for titration of effect. Its limitations are that circumferential flow is not achieved in Schlemm's canal and reduction of IOP is limited by episcleral venous pressure.

The procedure can be performed alone or easily combined with cataract surgery. The probe is inserted into the anterior chamber through a clear corneal incision after placement of viscoelastic. Under gonioscopic visualization, the probe is placed against the TM and 8 to 10 laser punctures are performed, spaced evenly across one quadrant. During the ablation, TM whitening and bubble formation is typical, followed by minor reflux of blood through the newly created openings. It is thought that the gas formation may also serve to accomplish a pneumatic canaloplasty and further enhance outflow. The probe is then withdrawn and the viscoelastic removed.

Due to lack of FDA approval, published clinical data on ELT have been largely from European studies where it has been approved since 1998. In 2006, Wilmsmeyer et al published results of their pilot study assessing the efficacy of ELT performed alone and ELT plus cataract surgery.[4] Success was defined as IOP of < 21 mm Hg and IOP reduction of at least 20%. Of the 69 patients receiving ELT alone, success was achieved in 60% at 6 months and 46% at 2 years. In the ELT plus cataract group, the success rate was higher at 85% at 6 months and 66% at 2 years. They did not report any serious laser-related complications. Safety and efficacy was further evaluated in another study of 21 patients undergoing ELT for open-angle glaucoma.[5] After a follow-up of over 2 years, mean IOP was reduced by 31.8%. While over 90% of patients received an IOP reduction of 20% or more, 38.1% of these required additional medical therapy. No clinically significant complications were reported. Finally, another study reported 1-year results in 28 open-angle glaucoma patients undergoing combined ELT and cataract surgery.[6] IOP was significantly lowered by a mean of 34.7% while number of glaucoma medications were reduced by a mean of 0.79.

In a prospective, randomized trial, Babighian et al compared ELT versus SLT treatment over 180 degrees of angle.[7] A total of 30 consecutive patients were followed for 2 years after treatment. Patients randomized to ELT received 8 laser spots while patients in the SLT group received 50 laser spots across 180 degrees of the angle. Success was defined as an IOP reduction of at least 20% without further intervention. The complete success rate was 53.3% in the ELT group, and 40% in the SLT group, although the difference failed to reach statistical significance. Mean IOP in the ELT group decreased from 25.0 to 17.6 mm Hg (29.6% reduction), while IOP in the SLT group decreased from 23.9 to 19.1 mm Hg (21% reduction). ELT complications included only a slight and transient anterior chamber bleeding after laser treatment in addition to a transient and mild IOP increase immediately postoperatively.

Scleral Spacing/Implants

The concept of scleral spacing with the PresView Scleral Implant (PSI, Refocus Group, Inc, Dallas, TX) was initially developed as a means of surgically correcting presbyopia. The polymethyl methacrylate micro-implants were designed to be implanted within the sclera as a means of lifting or vaulting the sclera overlying the ciliary muscle. This vaulting would in theory increase the distance between the ciliary muscle and lens, restoring lost tension on zonules to restore accommodation. During trials of the device, an IOP-lowering effect of about 20% was also noticed on normotensive presbyopes receiving the devices. The exact mechanism of IOP reduction in this procedure is unknown. The proposed mechanism of action stems from the stretching along the equator to tighten the ciliary muscle/zonule/lens complex and provide a resultant pulling effect on the scleral spur to open the TM and facilitate aqueous outflow. A biochemical remodeling effect is also proposed through metalloproteinase production in the angle.

The procedure requires a conjunctival dissection to access the 4 oblique quadrants of bare sclera in between the recti muscles. Four intrascleral tunnels are then constructed in a circular arrangement just posterior to the equator using a specially designed scleratome. Each lamellar scleral tunnel measures approximately 4-mm long, 1.5-mm wide, and 400-microns deep. The PSI is then inserted into the tunnel and locked into place with its adjoining piece.

Although no published clinical results of this procedure are available yet, 4-year outcomes have been presented from a Canadian study recently.[8] In this pilot study by Soloway, 24 eyes with ocular hypertension or open-angle glaucoma taking 1 to 3 medications were enrolled and underwent the procedure. At 1 year, mean IOP reduction was 20% with a mean reduction in medication use by 1.3 agents. Fifty-six percent of patients achieved IOP control without medication at this time point. By 48 months, 50% of eyes continued off medications and maintained IOP control. Medication use was reduced in 78% of patients.

Advantages of this procedure include its minimally invasive, nonpenetrating nature and potential to restore accommodation concurrently. The main disadvantages of PSI for glaucoma treatment include the need for conjunctival dissection and placement of scleral implants in all 4 quadrants, which can potentially interfere with future surgery. With limited evidence thus far, much more information on the efficacy and safety of the device is clearly needed. Clinical trials are currently ongoing in the United States and Europe.

InnFocus MicroShunt

While traditional glaucoma drainage devices are certainly not contained in the realm of MIGS, the novel InnFocus MicroShunt (Innovia LLC, Miami, FL) was designed as a minimally invasive drainage implant. Compared to traditional drainage implants, the InnFocus MicroShunt does not contain a large attached plate and is made of the novel compound poly(styrene-block-isobutylene-block-styrene) or SIBS. SIBS has been found to be a very biostable compound that does not oxidize or hydrolyze in the body and was shown to be significantly less inflammatory compared to silicone in rabbit eyes.[9] The microtube is still inserted into the anterior chamber from an ab externo approach and allows diversion of aqueous fluid to a subconjunctival bleb (Figure 11-3). The microtube is 9.5 mm in length with a 50- to 70-μm lumen diameter. Two small, attached fins are wedged into a scleral pocket to prevent migration. The flexibility of the tube allows it to conform to the contour of the globe upon implantation.

Preclinical evaluation of the device was initially described by Acosta et al in 2006.[9] The SIBS implant was placed in 16 eyes of New Zealand white rabbits and compared to silicone implants of similar shape. At 6 months, a low diffuse bleb was present along with tube patency in all SIBS implants. Good biocompatibility was noted with less encapsulation compared to silicone implants. Immunostaining of tissue surrounding the silicone implants showed collagen deposition and myofibroblast differentiation while the tissue surrounding the SIBS implants had no macrophages or myofibroblasts present. More recently, another study looked at biocompatibility of SIBS drainage implants in rabbit eyes across differing lumen sizes.[10] Mild chronic inflammation was noted around the tube at 6 months but no serious complications occurred. When comparing lumen sizes, there was no IOP difference; however, the smaller lumen size of 70 μm demonstrated fewer complications.

Initial clinical use of the InnFocus MicroShunt implant has been promising. Batile et al recently presented a cohort of 23 eyes undergoing InnFocus MicroShunt implantation with (n = 9) or without phacoemulsification (n = 14).[11] Intraoperative mitomycin C was also applied intraoperatively for 3 minutes at a concentration of 0.4 mg/mL. At a mean follow-up time of 11.2 months, IOP was lowered by 50% with the implant alone, and 64% when combined with cataract surgery. Complete success, defined as IOP ≤ 21 mm Hg or IOP reduction ≥ 20% without medical therapy, was reached in 86% and qualified success (same criteria with medications) was achieved in 100% of patients. Two cases of transient hypotony were reported along with 2 cases of choroidal effusions,

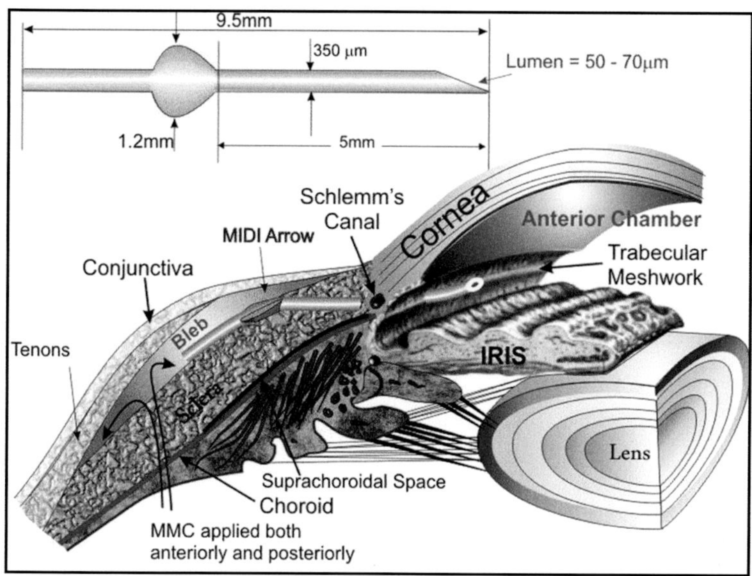

Figure 11-3. The InnFocus MicroShunt. The flexible implant is 9.5-mm long with 2 fins positioned 5 mm from the anterior chamber end to provide stabilization. The tube is inserted into the anterior chamber to divert aqueous fluid to a subconjunctival bleb. (Reprinted with permission from Innovia LLC.)

which spontaneously resolved. Mean postoperative IOP in patients receiving the implant alone was 11.1 mm Hg.

Transciliary Filtration

The Fugo blade (Medisurg Research and Management Corp, Norristown, PA) is an electrosurgical device that utilizes plasma energy to achieve precise tissue cutting on the eye both internally and externally. Tissue incisions are created with noncauterizing hemostasis and minimal collateral tissue damage. A microscopic plasma cloud is formed around a filament at the device tip that dissolves molecular bonds of the target tissue. The instrument has been used for capsulorrhexis, pupillary membrane removal, surgical iridotomy, and pediatric eye disease. The instrument can also be utilized to generate a transciliary filtration pathway to lower IOP. The procedure is designed to create external filtration of aqueous from the posterior chamber to the subconjunctival space.

In transciliary filtration, a conjunctival flap is made to expose the anterior sclera. Next, the 600-μm tip of the Fugo blade is used to make a full-thickness scleral pit approximately 1 mm^2 in area overlying the ciliary body. A smaller tip (100 or 300 μm) is then placed into this scleral window to create an opening through the pars plicata into the posterior chamber. Mitomycin C may then be placed to limit postoperative scarring, and the conjunctiva is reapproximated to the limbus. Pilocarpine is used for several weeks to avoid iris incarceration into the opening. A transconjunctival variation on this procedure has been described where the conjunctiva is moved anteriorly, and a 300-μm Fugo tip is used to pass through conjunctiva, sclera, and ciliary body into the posterior chamber.

The theoretic advantages of transciliary filtration are the posterior route of aqueous filtration, relatively low cost, and shorter surgery time relative to trabeculectomy. The disadvantages are that it is still a full-thickness external filtration procedure with resultant bleb formation. Thus, complications such as overfiltration and hypotony are still possible.

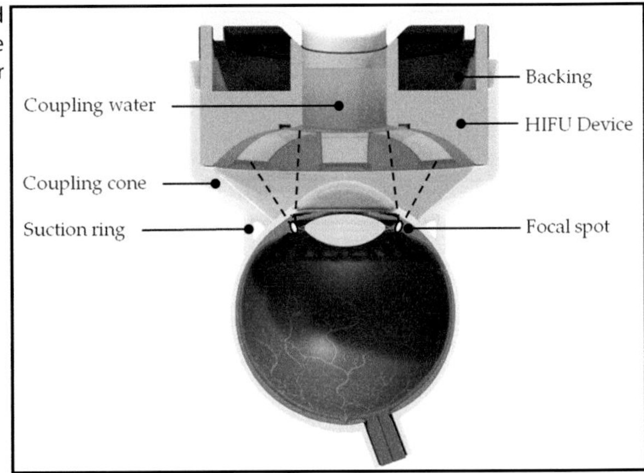

Figure 11-4. HIFU device. The suction ring and coupling cone are fitted to the surface of the eye. Miniaturized piezoelectric transducers deliver HIFU energy to the ciliary processes.

Limited clinical trials of this procedure have been published to date. The first report of transciliary filtration with the Fugo blade was a retrospective study of 147 cases with only 6 months of follow-up.[12] Success was defined as IOP < 21 mm Hg without medications or need for further surgery. While specific IOP data were not available in the report, success was achieved in 125 patients (85%). In a nonrandomized, prospective case series by Dow and deVeneci, 60 eyes of 36 consecutive patients with glaucoma underwent transciliary filtration.[13] Success was achieved in 76.6% of eyes at 6 months of follow-up; however, this was generously defined at IOP < 30 mm Hg without medication.

High Intensity Focused Ultrasound

High intensity focused ultrasound (HIFU) is a new way of achieving an old method of IOP reduction in glaucoma. Destruction of the ciliary body has been achieved in the past by cryotherapy and photocoagulation with a number of different laser modalities. Another method of treatment studied in the 1980s and 1990s was ultrasonic heating and destruction of tissue using HIFU.[14-16] The procedure has some inherent advantages in that energy can pass through nonoptical portions of the eye yet still be focused precisely within the target tissue. Targeting of energy is not dependent on pigmentation of tissue like diode laser therapy. The procedure was demonstrated effective in the past, but was largely abandoned due to the bulk of transducers and the time and complexity involved with the procedure. A newer and much smaller piezoelectric transducer is now available with the EyeOP1 system (EyeTechCare, Rillieux la Pape, France). These miniaturized transducers convert electrical energy into high frequency mechanical vibration. The high frequency ultrasound is focused precisely within the ciliary body, resulting in coagulation of the tissue by hyperthermia. Tissues immediately surrounding the target are left essentially unaffected.

The procedure can be accomplished in a noninvasive manner under local anesthesia. A ring-shaped therapy probe containing 6 active piezoelectric elements is inserted into a coupling cone that is held on the surface of the eye by suction (Figure 11-4). The cone and probe are connected to a command module containing the power generator and suction along with controls to customize treatment. Each of the 6 transducers has a segment measuring 10.2 mm in radius, 4.5 mm in width, and 7 mm in length (surface area of about 35 mm^2).[17] The HIFU energy is delivered from each transducer in succession to create a circumferential treatment within the ciliary body. The procedure has the advantages of being titratable, noninvasive, and repeatable. Potential disadvantages mirror those of established methods of cyclodestruction, including hypotony, inflammation, and phthisis.

Preclinical evaluation of HIFU was published by Aptel et al in 2010.[18] In this study, 18 eyes of 18 rabbits were treated using a ring composed of 6 sector transducers. Eyes were divided into 1 of 3 groups, with group 1 receiving treatment from all sectors, group 2 receiving treatment from 5, and group 3 receiving treatment from only 4 at 2 watts of power. At 28 days posttreatment, IOP was reduced by 28.1% in group 3, 25.5% in group 2, and 55.3% in group 1. Inflammation was reported as limited and no obvious anterior segment abnormalities were noted. Histologic analysis showed well-demarcated coagulative necrosis within the ciliary body without damage to the lens or sclera.

The first clinical pilot study was completed in 2011 in France.[17] In this prospective, noncontrolled study 12 eyes of 12 patients with refractory glaucoma and uncontrolled IOP were treated with HIFU using 6 transducers. A power setting of 2 W was used for all patients, but the duration of each pulse varied from 3 seconds in group 1 (n = 4) to 4 seconds in group 2 (n = 8). Patients were followed by clinical exam and ultrasound biomicroscopy (UBM) evaluation of anterior segment structures. After 6 months of follow-up, IOP was reduced in group 1 eyes from a mean preoperative IOP of 35.6 to 27.1 mm Hg postoperatively. Medication use decreased from a mean of 2.5 medications to 2.3 after the procedure. In group 2, mean preoperative IOP decreased from 40.5 to 23.4 mm Hg after treatment with medications modestly increasing from 3.3 to 3.5. No major intraoperative or postoperative complications were reported. Self-limited superficial corneal disease was noted in 4 patients, all of whom had pre-existing corneal pathology. UBM studies showed focal and reproducible cystic involution of ciliary processes without collateral damage. Suprachoroidal fluid collections were noted in 6 of 12 eyes. Further clinical trials of HIFU are currently ongoing to better characterize this treatment.

Conclusion

The recent surge in development of MIGS devices and novel approaches to surgically treat glaucoma has produced many exciting approaches for use in the operating room today and in the near future. As with any new approach, clinical data are still evolving and the true efficacy of these new procedures will need to be better understood and quantified. What is exciting, however, is that the glaucoma surgeon currently has many options at his or her disposal to tailor therapies for each patient. These options are increasing and will allow for improved individualized care for patients moving forward.

References

1. Pajic B, Pajic-Eggspuehler B, Haefliger I. New minimally invasive, deep sclerotomy ab interno surgical procedure for glaucoma, six years of follow-up. *J Glaucoma.* 2011;20(2):109-114.
2. Merula R, Haefliger, IO, Cronemberger, S, et. al. The influence of thalamosinusotomy under different constant intraocular pressures on aqueous outflow facility in isolated porcine eyes. *Rev Bras Oftalmol.* 2008;67:12-18.
3. Francis BA, Singh K, Lin SC, et al. Novel glaucoma procedures: a report by the American Academy of Ophthalmology. *Ophthalmology.* 2011;118:1466-1480.
4. Wilmsmeyer S, Philippin H, Funk J. Excimer laser trabeculotomy: a new, minimally invasive procedure for patients with glaucoma. *Graefes Arch Clin Exp Ophthalmol.* 2006;244(6):670-676.
5. Babighian S, Rapizzi E, Galan A. Efficacy and safety of ab interno excimer laser trabeculotomy in primary open-angle glaucoma: two years of follow-up. *Ophthalmologica.* 2006;220(5):285-290.
6. Töteberg-Harms M, Ciechanowski PP, Hirn C, Funk J. One-year results after combined cataract surgery and excimer laser trabeculotomy for elevated intraocular pressure [in German]. *Ophthalmologe.* 2011;108:733-738.
7. Babighian S, Caretti L, Tavolato M, Cian R, Galan A. Excimer laser trabeculotomy vs 180 degrees selective laser trabeculoplasty in primary open-angle glaucoma. A 2-year randomized, controlled trial. *Eye (Lond).* 2010;24(4):632-638.

8. Soloway BaR, Aaron. Scleral spacing procedure and its indication in glaucoma treatment. *Ophthalmology Times Europe*. 2011.
9. Acosta AC, Espana EM, Yamamoto H, et al. A newly designed glaucoma drainage implant made of poly(styrene-b-isobutylene-b-styrene): biocompatibility and function in normal rabbit eyes. *Arch Ophthalmol.* 2006;124(12):1742-1749.
10. Arrieta EA, Aly M, Parrish R, et al. Clinicopathologic correlations of poly-(styrene-b-isobutylene-b-styrene) glaucoma drainage devices of different internal diameters in rabbits. *Ophthalmic Surg Lasers Imaging.* 2011;42(4):338-345.
11. Batile J, Fantes, F, Alburquerque, R, et al. One year follow-up of a novel minimally invasive glaucoma drainage implant. American Academy of Ophthalmology Annual Meeting. 2012; Abstract.
12. Singh D, Singh, K. Transciliary filtraion using the Fugo Blade. *Ann Ophthalmol (Skokie).* 2002;34:183-187.
13. Dow CT, deVenecia G. Transciliary filtration (Singh filtration) with the Fugo plasma blade. *Ann Ophthalmol (Skokie).* 2008;40:8-14.
14. Coleman DJ, Lizzi FL, Driller J, et al. Therapeutic ultrasound in the treatment of glaucoma. II. Clinical applications. *Ophthalmology.* 1985;92(3):347-353.
15. Coleman DJ, Lizzi FL, Driller J, et al. Therapeutic ultrasound in the treatment of glaucoma. I. Experimental model. *Ophthalmology.* 1985;92(3):339-346.
16. Maskin SL, Mandell AI, Smith JA, Wood RC, Terry SA. Therapeutic ultrasound for refractory glaucoma: a three-center study. *Ophthalmic Surg.* 1989;20(3):186-192.
17. Aptel F, Charrel T, Lafon C, et al. Miniaturized high-intensity focused ultrasound device in patients with glaucoma: a clinical pilot study. *Invest Ophthalmol Vis Sci.* 2011;52(12):8747-8753.
18. Aptel F, Charrel T, Palazzi X, Chapelon JY, Denis P, Lafon C. Histologic effects of a new device for high-intensity focused ultrasound cyclocoagulation. *Invest Ophthalmol Vis Sci.* 2010;51(10):5092-5098.

12

Future Directions in Glaucoma Therapeutic Devices and Treatment Approaches

Sean Ianchulev, MD, MPH and Sarwat Salim, MD, FACS

In previous chapters, we discussed new emerging devices and surgical approaches to treating glaucoma, including minimally invasive glaucoma surgical innovation, microstents, and other surgical techniques for enhanced trabecular and nontrabecular aqueous outflow. Many of these approaches are in advanced clinical stages of development or have already been approved in different countries, such as the European Union, for surgical use. Here we would like to look beyond the immediate therapeutic horizon of innovation to explore novel approaches, technology trends, and transformational science that are likely to impact the future glaucoma treatment landscape. Where are the unmet needs, and what technologies are being actively developed to address them? While it is hard to predict the future direction and success of innovation, our goal is to reach through the "keyhole" of innovation to palpate the current trends in preclinical and clinical investigation that create the platform for potential leapfrog developments and breakthrough devices in the future.

Drug Delivery Techniques and Sustained Release Implants

Drug delivery continues to be one of the greatest unmet needs and challenges in glaucoma treatment. The need is obvious—glaucoma is a chronic, life-long disease that requires self-administered, daily treatment with one or multiple medications. Adherence to medical therapy is very poor, and there is a big gap between prescribed regimens and what the patient actually does on a daily basis. Despite many new pharmaceuticals with optimized therapeutic profiles, we are still limited to daily topical eyedrop administration and delivery, which have changed little over the past 100 years. Currently, more than 90% of ophthalmic drugs are delivered through eyedrops, which are inefficient due to rapid tear turnover and drug absorption in the conjunctiva. Because eyedrops are rapidly cleared and limited by corneal bioavailability of about 1% to 5%, overdosing and frequent administration are required to maintain the drug concentration within the therapeutic range. In today's patient-centric and outcomes-driven clinical world, the need for an alternative to daily eyedrops cannot be more obvious.

Kahook MY.
MIGS: Advances in Glaucoma Surgery (pp 101-116).

A number of devices and drug-device combinations are focusing on this problem, and new technology and capabilities are presenting exciting development opportunities that were not previously available. In terms of drug delivery and sustained release, advances in nanotechnology and polymer science, coupled with minimally invasive intervention for less traumatic and safer implantation and access to the ocular anatomy, are likely to solve the long-standing problems associated with controlling the pharmacokinetics of drug release to achieve more clinically meaningful therapeutic windows of retreatment. It should be noted that drug delivery is a major problem not only in glaucoma but also in the treatment of retinal diseases, such as macular degeneration and diabetic retinopathy. Therefore, recent advances in biologic therapies have changed the treatment paradigm, and many of these therapies now require monthly intravitreal injection. Parallel to the needs in glaucoma, this drives significant research efforts to find better ways to deliver ocular therapies, which will invariably spill over and help the innovation process for sustained delivery of glaucoma therapeutics.

Punctal Plugs

Several approaches for sustained drug delivery of glaucoma medications are being investigated. Probably farthest along in development is the punctal plug technology.[1,2] Punctal plugs, long used to treat dry eye syndrome, decrease tear drainage by blocking the nasolacrimal duct. The duration of this blockage varies with the type of material composing the plug, with those made from animal collagen on the shorter end (7 to 10 days), and those made from synthetic materials, such as silicone, Teflon (Du Pont, Ontario, Canada), hydroxyethyl metacrylate (HEM), polycaprolactone (PCL), or polydioxanone retaining their occlusive properties for up to 6 months.[1] Potential advantages of punctal plugs relative to eyedrops include minimization of side effects because a lower quantity of drug is required, better control of intraocular pressure (IOP) because of controlled release of the drug, and improved patient compliance. Failure of punctal plugs is typically due to spontaneous extrusion, which appears to be more common when the plug is inserted into the upper rather than the lower punctum. Retention rates as low as 50% over a single month are not uncommon. Polymers that give the plug better retention properties, such as the thermosensitive acrylic polymer used in the SmartPlug (Medennium, Inc, Irvine, CA) or the Shape Memory Polymer Plug (Shape Ophthalmics LLC, Denver, CO), are being developed to address this problem. For use as a drug delivery system, the body of the punctal plug is typically coated with a material that cannot be permeated by either the drug or the tear film. Drug contained in the polymeric core is released from the uncoated head of the plug and passively diffuses into the tear film. Some types of plugs are instead coated with a drug-containing polymeric matrix or soaked in a drug solution, although this approach may result in a reduced amount of the drug being delivered. Most types of plugs achieve near zero-order drug release rates for the drug that is loaded into the device.

Two punctal plug devices that have advanced to Phase 2 trials are the Latanoprost Punctal Plug Delivery System (L-PPDS) being developed by QLT, Inc (Vancouver, BC, Canada) and the OTX-TP2 plug for delivery of sustained-release travoprost (Ocular Therapeutix, Inc, Bedford, MA). In October 2008, QLT announced results of the CORE study, a 12-week, Phase 2, randomized, double-masked, parallel-group, multicenter trial of the safety and preliminary efficacy of 3 dose levels of latanoprost (3.5, 14, and 21 μg) delivered by the L-PPDS in 61 patients with open-angle glaucoma (OAG) or ocular hypertension (OHT) and a mean baseline IOP of 24 mm Hg. Statistically significant reductions from baseline IOP ranging from 3.2 to 5.2 mm Hg were achieved at weeks 4, 8, and 12.[3] The overall adverse events ranged from 1.6% to 14.8%, with increased tear production and mild, transient ocular discomfort as the most common complaints. Neither IOP reduction nor adverse event rates were dose dependent. Additional Phase 2 studies using substantially higher latanoprost doses are under way.[1] Preliminary results with 44-μg L-PPDS administered to 60 patients demonstrated a mean reduction from baseline IOP of 3.5 mm Hg at week 4, with an IOP drop of ≥ 5 mm Hg in 36% of patients. The majority of patients (78%) retained the plug in both eyes for 4 weeks, with an overall adverse event rate of 1.7% to 11.7%, with increased tear production, ocular discomfort, and eye itchiness and irritation as the most common complaints. In October 2012, Ocular Therapeutix announced results of a 2-month pilot Phase 2 study evaluating the OTX-TP2 in 20 patients (36 eyes) with OAG or OHT and a baseline IOP of ≥ 24 mm Hg (mean, 29 mm Hg).[4] Reductions in mean IOP were 7.2 mm Hg after 2 weeks and were still at 6.8 mm Hg after 8 weeks. The QLT Plug drug delivery system is now under development by MATI Therapeutics.

The efficacy profile of punctal plugs looks promising, and the devices appear to be well tolerated overall. However, additional and longer-term studies are needed to address the problems of device extrusion, excessive lacrimation, ocular discomfort, and the potential for bacterial accumulation due to punctal occlusion, which in some cases may lead to canaliculitis.[2,5]

Contact Lenses

Another approach to sustained delivery to the ocular surface is the use of contact lenses as a drug elution vehicle.[1,2,6] With more than 38 million contact lens wearers in the United States alone, and with several decades of clinical experience, it is obvious why contact lenses are acutely targeted as a drug delivery approach. Because of the affinity of hydrogel materials for water-soluble drugs, bandage contact lenses can be used as depots to elute glaucoma medications, anti-inflammatories, and anti-infective agents, among others. Traditionally, lenses were loaded with drugs by presoaking the lens in the active medication to achieve the effect of a depot that can release the drug slowly over time. Results with this approach have been inconsistent due to variability of drug solubility, drug elution rates, lens material properties, and other factors.[1]

Material science in hydrogel development continues to evolve, and adding adjuncts such as silicone to conventional hydrogel materials[7] has been demonstrated to improve permeability and ocular bioavailability of medications beyond what can be achieved by eyedrops.[1,2] Numerous novel techniques have been used to extend the pharmacokinetics of delivery with contact lenses.[1,2] Among them are drug liposome encapsulation,[8-11] incorporation of drug particles and nanoparticles directly into the lens material,[12,13] use of polymer and fibrin films,[14] lens-incorporated cyclodextrins,[1,15] and adding surfactants to control drug release.[1,15] Imprinting of drugs onto contact lenses,[16-18] incorporating transport barriers, and impregnating the drug within the lens matrix by use of solvents are some alternative approaches being tried.[15]

The study of contact lenses for drug delivery dates back to 1960, when Wichterle first demonstrated this clinical application.[19] Currently, there is no FDA-approved product for contact lens-based drug delivery, but given the latest advances in material science, this could change very soon.

External Pumps

Several innovative technologies using miniature external pumps are currently in preclinical development.[2] For example, the Replenish, Inc (Pasadena, CA) pump system is a nonabsorbed, semipermanent device composing a drug reservoir, a hydrolysis-based pump system, and a transscleral cannula for drug delivery into the anterior or posterior chamber.[20] The reservoir is implanted under the conjunctiva, and the cannula is placed through an incision in the anterior or posterior segment. The rate of drug delivery is controlled by a 1-way check valve in the pump. Because the reservoir is refillable in place, the device can theoretically be used for drug delivery over a period of years. The Replenish device and other manually and electrically controlled miniature drug pumps typically exploit the principles of Micro-Electro-Mechanical Systems (MEMS). Second-generation devices include an electrolysis pump that is separated from the drug reservoir and integrated valves for controlled, programmable drug delivery. Bolus and continuous pumping, as well as variation in the drug-flow rate, will be possible. Clinical studies are needed to determine the efficacy and safety of this new technology. Refillability allows long-term use with added advantage, but it also raises concerns about the potential for infection and the need for sterile technique.

Subconjunctival Injections/Inserts

Conjunctival or subconjunctival administration of IOP-lowering agents is another approach for sustained release over a 3- to 4-month interval—a time frame that approximates the frequency of routine clinic visits for glaucoma management.[2,15] The objective here is to match the degradation rates of biocompatible and biodegradable polymers under the conjunctival space. The challenge with this approach is conjunctival scarring and trauma from repeated injections. Also, scleral permeability and interaction with the physicochemical drug properties (hydrophilicity/lipophilicity) have been particularly challenging. Subconjunctival injection of hydrophilic drugs that penetrate the sclera is generally more successful than injection of water-soluble drugs, as diffusion across the conjunctival epithelium is a significant rate-limiting factor for the latter.[15]

A few subconjunctival approaches to drug delivery are currently in early-stage development. A latanoprost-releasing subconjunctival implant being collaboratively developed by Pfizer and pSivida is in Phase I/II clinical trials at the University of Kentucky.[21] Also, a latanoprost-releasing insert (Aerie Pharmaceuticals, Bridgewater, NJ) is being studied preclinically. Little data are available for this approach to ophthalmic drug delivery.

Intravitreal Inserts/Implants

Biodegradable and nonbiodegradable polymer intravitreal implants are being investigated for drug delivery to the back of the eye, and 3 are currently approved for indications other than glaucoma (Vitrasert [Bausch & Lomb, Rochester, NY], Retisert [Bausch & Lomb], and Ozurdex [Allergan, Irvine, CA]).[1] While degradable implants offer the advantage of eventual clearance of all system components from the eye over time, they are less efficient in releasing drugs in a precisely controlled fashion than are the nondegradable versions that ultimately require surgical removal when their drug loads are depleted.

Potential advantages of both types of intravitreal implants over the conventionally used drug delivery systems include delivery of the drug closer to target tissues in the posterior segment and minimization of side effects due to a lower dose requirement. Challenges include the possibility of burst release of the drugs under some circumstances.

Of the 3 currently approved intravitreal implants, only the Ozurdex implant is biodegradable. As is typical of biodegradable implants, this one is made of a polymer that is degraded to water and carbon dioxide in the body. Allergan is currently developing a brimonidine tartrate-releasing implant on the Ozurdex PLGA polymer platform. The same platform might apply to other glaucoma therapeutic categories.

Suprachoroidal Delivery

The suprachoroidal space (SCS) has been a therapeutic target for drug delivery for many years, but only now do we have the tools to allow us to access it with minimally invasive interventional approaches. Unlike the intravitreal space, the SCS does not impinge on the visual axis and is better suited as a sustained-release drug depot to both the posterior and anterior segments. As such, it can be used to deliver therapeutics for diseases such as age-related macular degeneration and glaucoma. More importantly, this dual access to the posterior and anterior segment can be critical in the future when neuroprotective or stem-cell agents enter the therapeutic paradigm.

Microneedles and microcannulation can now access the SCS, and initial experience demonstrates that volumes of 50 to 100 μL can safely be injected.[22] Initial studies show comparative advantages over intravitreal delivery.[23] In one study, a microneedle SCS delivery method was directly compared with intravitreal delivery of fluorescein, fluorescently tagged dextrans

(40 and 250 kDa), bevacizumab, and polymeric particles (20 nm and 10 μm diameter) in vivo in rabbits.[24] Patel et al demonstrated that the SCS route achieved a 10-fold higher concentration of the injected material in the back of the eye than in the anterior tissues, whereas there was no significant posterior versus anterior segment selectivity with intravitreal injection.[24] Half-life of the particles injected into the SCS depended on size; those with molecular weight of 0.3 to 250 kDA had a half-life from 1.2 to 7.9 h, but particles ranging from 20 nm to 10 μm had not cleared the eye after a period of months and were still detected primarily in the SCS and choroid.

Evidence obtained using a flexible fiberoptic microcannula for injecting drugs into the SCS in pigs suggested that this route may prove to be more practical for delivery of small molecules than for larger biological molecules,[25] presumably because of the collagen matrix of the scleral tissue.[26] In a 2006 study, Olsen et al demonstrated in a porcine model that microcannulation of the SCS delivered a small molecule, triamcinolone in a sustained-release matrix, to the macula for at least 120 days.[27] In their 2011 study, Olsen et al compared the pharmacokinetics and tissue response to the macromolecule bevacizumab when injected via the typical intravitreal route versus the SCS route.[25] Bevacizumab had a more sustained pharmacologic profile when delivered intravitreally and achieved more direct distribution to the inner retinal tissues than when delivered via the SCS route. The investigators concluded that sustained-release formulations should be considered for optimizing delivery of larger biological molecules via the SCS pathway.

Pilot studies of suprachoroidal drug delivery of triamcinolone and/or bevacizumab via a microcatheter have been performed in patients with advanced macular disease and/or who have not responded to conventional therapies.[28] Pathologies treated in these studies included choroidal neovascularization secondary to exudative age-related macular degeneration and retinal vein occlusion or diffuse diabetic macular edema accompanied by subfoveal hard exudates. These small studies have provided encouraging results, including some increase in residual vision and significant reduction of macular edema without surgical complications or unmanageable postoperative adverse events.

If larger, prospective clinical trials support the promising results obtained in the animal models and human pilot studies, it is expected that delivery of drugs via the SCS would offer several advantages over conventional drug delivery methods used to target the back of the eye. As noted by Patel et al,[29] the 4 characteristics desirable for effective drug delivery to the posterior segment include (1) the procedure be minimally invasive and safe, (2) the procedure should effectively target the desired tissues with limited exposure to the drug in other ocular regions, (3) sustained drug exposure should be possible so that repetition of the procedure is minimized and better therapeutic control is achieved, and (4) the procedure should be sufficiently simple so that it can be performed at a routine office visit. Delivery of drugs via the uveoscleral route has the potential to meet all of these criteria. Moreover, a recent study in a rabbit model demonstrated that the SCS can be used for virally vectored gene delivery—potentially a less invasive and safer method than currently used procedures for gene delivery in eyes with hereditary pathologies, such as Leber's congenital amaurosis.[30]

Drug-Coated Glaucoma Stents and Implants

With the advent of minimally invasive glaucoma surgical implants and stents (iStent [Glaukos Corp, Laguna Hills, CA], CyPass Micro-Stent [Transcend Medical, Menlo Park, CA], Hydrus Microstent [Ivantis Inc, Irvine, CA], AqueSys [AqueSys, Irvine, CA]), the opportunity for sustained intraocular drug elution is on the horizon. While no drug-coated stents are in clinical development at this time, some companies are considering and developing drug elution approaches in combination with microstents and shunts that are likely to follow the clinical experience with some of the drug-eluting cardiac stents.

Topical Drug Delivery Microdroplet Sprays

While most approaches discussed previously try to eliminate or replace the use of daily topical administration, there are alternative technologies that attempt to improve it. The eyedropper has significant limitations, and multiple studies have documented these shortcomings.[1,2,15] Most patients have difficulty administering eyedrops, and many cannot administer them directly into their eye. Dripping, spillage, and overflow are some of the day-to-day practical issues that hinder patient use and compliance. Overdosing is another problem; the capacity of an eye drop is about 27 μL, which well exceeds the 7- to 8-μL holding capacity of the ocular surface and cul de sac. Furthermore, uneven distribution and retention to the ocular surface, as well as low intraocular bioavailability (1% to 5%), are some of the fundamental challenges for all topical formulations.

Microdroplet collimated sprays are currently in development (Corinthian Ophthalmics, Inc, Raleigh, NC) as an alternative to conventional eyedrops. Key to this new approach is the ability to control droplet size consistently to eliminate flow turbulence, air drag, and evaporation typical of the regular atomizer sprays. This technology is leading to the creation of a collimated flow that can be administered in a rapid directional microjet to deliver the formulation onto the ocular surface at a speed 3 times faster than the blink rate. Recently presented clinical data[31] showed that a 6-μL microdroplet spray of phenylephrine 2.5% and tropicamide 1% achieved equivalent dilation to one eye drop (27 μL) of each drug. Preclinical studies of IOP-lowering agents in glaucomatous beagle dogs[31] showed similar equivalent results between eyedrops and microdroplet spray of one-quarter to one-fifth the amount of the same drug formulation in terms of IOP-lowering effect. The ability to efficiently deliver smaller but biologically equivalent quantities of the same formulation is critical for any formulation with preservatives, as it can reduce the exposure of the ocular surface and minimize untoward ocular effects. Such piezoelectric collimated microdroplet sprays also show promise for preservative-free multi-dosing, as the sterility barriers and fluid ejection mechanisms prevent bacterial contamination of the liquid.

Devices for Monitoring Intraocular Pressure

Multiple studies have documented the imperfection of how we clinically measure IOP. IOP fluctuates significantly diurnally, yet in clinical practice we measure IOP at a single time point.[32] While in clinical studies it is advisable and often standard practice to measure diurnal IOP at a minimum of 3 time points, this is impractical in the setting of a busy clinical practice. In fact, almost 100% of diagnostic and monitoring IOP measurements in the clinic today are single-point measurements, which provide a limited biometric snapshot.

Fortunately, new research and technology are paving the way for continuous IOP sensing by new microdevices with telebiometric processing. A number of technologies are in development. Sensimed's Triggerfish (Lausanne, Switzerland) is farthest along in clinical trials, with other companies' devices at various stages of development, such as AcuMEMS (Menlo Park, CA), Mesotec/Implandata (Hannover, Germany), Ziemer Contact Lens (Ziemer Ophthalmic Systems AG, Port, Switzerland), Ophtimalia Contact Lens (Paris, France), Dundee, Moorfields contact lens (London, UK), Tissot Medical (Le Locle, France), Assenti (Louisville, KY), BioMEMS (Lyon, France), and Launchpoint (Goleta, CA).

The Triggerfish device consists of a highly oxygen-permeable silicone soft contact lens consisting of 2 sensing-resistive strain gauges that are capable of recording circumferential changes in the area of the corneoscleral junction (Figure 12-1). The device senses changes in corneal curvature and circumference, which presumably correlate with IOP. A microprocessor embedded in the contact lens communicates wirelessly through a patched periorbital antenna that is connected to a portable recorder that the patient wears around the waist. The device can record IOP fluctuations up to 24 hours and remains active during undisturbed sleep. Three hundred data points are acquired during a 30-second measurement period, repeated every 5 minutes. The output of the

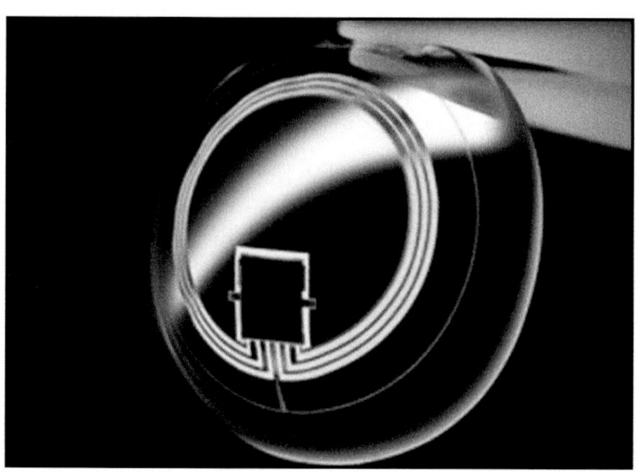

Figure 12-1. Triggerfish contact lens with antenna and strain gauge.

sensor is not in millimeters of mercury as with most conventional IOP applanation devices but in arbitrary electrical units that relate to the surface recording from the cornea in response to IOP fluctuations. The device is currently approved in Europe but not in the United States, and clinical validation studies are under way. In a recent study[33] of 40 patients, repeated use of the contact lens sensor demonstrated good safety and tolerability with fair to good reproducibility. Similar contact lens-based approaches are being developed by a number of other companies, including Ziemer and Ophtimalia.

Another device in development is an implantable IOP-sensing device called the iSense System (AcuMEMS, Inc). The iSense System uses implantable microelectromechanical systems (MEMS) sensors that couple to a hand-held reader, which enables wireless and direct IOP measurement. A dynamic IOP measurement system that allows IOP changes to be continuously tracked by the glaucoma patient and ophthalmologist is being developed. Implandata Ophthalmic Products is also developing a microsensor device that will continuously monitor IOP in an approach similar to the AcuMEMS, using a permanent sensor that is implanted and connected remotely to an external hand-held device. Two versions of the device will be available, one for intraocular placement in conjunction with cataract surgery and a second with extraocular placement for other patients.

The future of glaucoma devices will likely see many such IOP-sensing and telemonitoring approaches as microprocessor technology rapidly converges on the unmet need for better continuous IOP monitoring.

New Surgical Approaches

Stents and Shunts

We have discussed previously an array of new microstent approaches with minimally invasive implantation (eg, iStent, CyPass Micro-Stent, and Hydrus Microstent). These devices are in different stages of clinical development with the objective of demonstrating not only safety and efficacy but also the long-term duration of effect over a course of at least 2 years. This innovation will open up the field of minimally invasive glaucoma intervention and could transform the landscape of glaucoma treatment by introducing surgical procedures much earlier in the disease course, particularly in combination with phaco-cataract surgery.

For all of these technologies, it will be critical to control the wound-healing process over time to ensure sustained function and effect. Therefore, future developments for optimal stent configurations and approaches will likely focus on surface modification, material science, drug elution, and combinations of antifibrotic drug techniques.

Even before we see the clinical adoption of microstent technology, research on new materials is blazing a new trail in the footsteps of the MIGS devices.

The InnFocus MicroShunt (Innovia LLC, Miami, FL) uses a new material—poly(styrene-block-isobutylene-block-styrene) (SIBS)—that is currently being successfully used as the carrier for a drug-eluting coronary stent (TAXUS stent, Boston Scientific, Natick, MA).[34] SIBS is a biostable thermoplastic elastomer that shares some physical properties with silicone and polyurethane. However, it is the following properties that are making SIBS the subject of great interest to developers of stent and shunt devices: (1) it substantially activates platelets; (2) polymorphonuclear leukocytes are not typically seen in large numbers around SIBS implants; (3) clinically significant accumulation of myofibroblasts, scarring, and encapsulation are uncommon with SIBS-containing implants in the eye; (4) the implants do not become brittle over time; (5) calcification within the polymer does not occur; and (6) degradation of the material has yet to be seen in any living system. The biocompatibility of SIBS is hypothesized to be due to the inertness of the material and the absence of cleavable moieties that could attract phagocytes.

Research on a first-generation ophthalmic implant device using SIBS—the MIDI-Tube glaucoma shunt—was conducted by a team led by Jean-Marie Parel at the Bascom Palmer Eye Institute (University of Miami Miller School of Medicine) in conjunction with scientists at InnFocus.[35] The proximal end of the shunt was designed for insertion into the anterior chamber, bisecting the angle between the iris and cornea, with the distal end resting in a subconjunctival space/Tenon's flap created posterior to the limbus. A decrease in IOP results when aqueous humor drains from the anterior chamber into a bleb formed in the conjunctival flap and is then absorbed into the ocular venous system or through the conjunctiva into the tear ducts. As first reported in 2006,[35] a study in normal rabbit eyes showed that the MIDI-Tube shunt retained 100% patency 6 months after insertion, whereas a similarly designed silicone glaucoma drainage implant in control eyes induced collagen deposition and myofibroblast differentiation. No macrophages or myofibroblasts were seen in the tissue surrounding the SIBS implant. The authors concluded that SIBS shunts have the potential to decrease subconjunctival fibrosis that has been a problem with other implants, as well as to prevent postplacement hypotony. It has been noted, however, that this new material has its own potential limitations in clinical use, including creep deformation that might force SIBS into an undesirable shape and certain sterilization requirements.

The InnFocus MicroShunt, like the MIDI-Tube device, is a drainage implant composing a SIBS microtube inserted into the anterior chamber. It is currently being evaluated in 2 versions: one that shunts aqueous humor into the conjunctival bleb and another in which the tube is attached to a plate that both receives the shunted aqueous humor and also maintains the bleb. Clinical trials of the InnFocus MicroShunt are currently under way.

Lasers

Laser use is certainly not new in ophthalmology, dating back to the 1940s with photocoagulation of the retina and subsequently in the 1970s when Wise and Witter described the argon laser's use for treating the trabecular meshwork (TM).[36] Later, in the mid-1990s, Latina described the Q-switched frequency doubled Nd:YAG laser with short-pulse applications, now known as selective laser trabeculoplasty.[37]

Today, we are on the threshold of femtosecond (FS) laser evolution, with growing applications from cornea-refractive surgery to cataract surgery and now, not far behind, glaucoma surgery as well.[38] Since 2009 when Nagy et al described the use of an intraocular FS laser to perform capsulotomy and lens fragmentation in cataract surgery,[39]at least 3 devices have already been approved by the FDA for refractive cataract surgery. But this technology has other potential applications outside cataract and refractive surgery: namely, glaucoma surgery.[38] In 2005, Toyran et al tested the use of FS laser pulses to create fistulas in strips of human TM ex vivo, establishing a range of exposure times and energy dosages that might produce ablation channels in the TM without damaging the surrounding tissues.[40] In glaucomatous eyes, such channels might allow aqueous humor in the anterior chamber to directly access Schlemm's canal. In 2009, using a custom FS laser ablation system with a gonioscopic lens, Nakamura et al reported results of ex vivo studies in enucleated baboon eyes and human donor eyes that involved photodisruption of the TM.[41] Laser energy was directed toward the anterior chamber angle. Postsurgery, 2-photon microscopy revealed oblique, sharp-edged, trough-shaped lesions, with sparing of adjacent tissue and no thermal coagulation. Lesion dimensions increased linearly with both laser pulse energy and exposure time. If performed at the time of laser cataract surgery, this technique has the potential to allow simultaneous, minimally invasive treatment of TM obstruction in glaucomatous eyes.

Sclera-based glaucoma surgery using FS laser technology is also being investigated. In an early effort by Bahar and colleagues, reported in 2007,[42] superficial and deep partial-thickness scleral flaps were formed in human cadaveric eyes by the IntraLase FS laser (Abbot Medical Optics, Inc, Santa Ana, CA). Removal of the deep flap revealed percolation of aqueous humor through Descemet's window. Subsequently, using FS laser technology, Chai et al created partial-thickness drainage channels in the sclera of enucleated rabbit eyes and developed a 3-dimensional (3D) finite element model capable of predicting the effect of these channels on aqueous humor outflow and IOP.[43] Measurements in the perfused rabbit eyes showed that aqueous humor outflow increased following FS laser surgery. The 3D model predicted that, assuming a constant aqueous humor production rate, the effect of the laser-created channels would be an IOP reduction from 67% to 81%; the experimentally adjusted IOP values in the perfused rabbit eyes were in reasonable agreement with this prediction. The authors suggested that such a model could also be used to determine optimal channel dimension to achieve a specified increase in outflow facility and IOP reduction. A follow-up in vivo pilot study in rabbits, reported in 2010, demonstrated that partial-thickness subsurface drainage channels created in the sclera of experimental eyes by using an FS laser resulted in postoperative lowering of IOP compared with control eyes.[44] The magnitude of the IOP reduction increased as the dimensions of the channels increased.

These preclinical results are encouraging, but obstacles to clinical use of FS lasers include high cost and the need for intensive maintenance of the currently available FS laser platforms.[38] A combination of FS laser treatment for glaucoma with high-volume procedures, such as laser cataract ablation, has been suggested as one way of eventually reducing the price tag and making the procedure feasible in clinical practice.

CO_2 Laser-Assisted Sclerectomy

A different laser technology—CO_2 laser-assisted sclerectomy (CLASS)—holds promise as a surgical adjunct in conventional glaucoma surgery to improve precision and standardize surgical dissection in nonpenetrating deep sclerectomy. The self-controlled laser system ablates dry material (eg, the dry sclera) but is mostly absorbed by water. Scleral layers are ablated and removed until percolating fluid absorbs the energy, thereby attenuating further tissue ablation when the desired endpoint has been reached (Figure 12-2). In a multicenter, prospective study, Geffen et al[45] evaluated this technology using the OT-134-IOPtiMate (IOPtima Ltd, Ramat Gan, Israel) CO_2 laser system in 37 patients for whom primary filtration surgery was indicated for uncontrolled primary and pseudoexfoliative open-angle glaucoma. Thirty patients completed 12 months of follow-up. Complete success was defined as IOP ranging from 5 to 18 mm Hg and a 20% reduction from IOP baseline (mean baseline IOP = 26.3 mm Hg) with no medication at 12 months; qualified success was the same IOP range with medication. At 6 months, mean IOP had fallen to 14.4 mm Hg and at 12 months was 14.3 mm Hg, representing 42.4% and 40.7% reduction from baseline at 6 and 12 months, respectively ($P < 0.001$). At 6 months, 76.7% of patients had complete success and 83.3% had qualified success. At 12 months, complete success was achieved by 60% and qualified success by 86.6% of the patients. There were no laser-related complications; other complications were mild and transitory, resolving spontaneously or with conservative treatment within 1 month postsurgery. Following publication of the study, co-author Ehud Assia reported that the team had completed CLASS treatment in a series of 51 patients with IOP reduction from the baseline mean

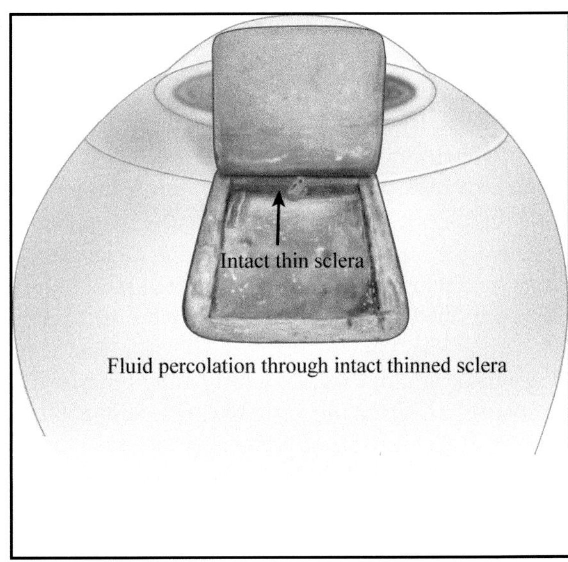

Figure 12-2. Laser-ablated sclera allows for egress of aqueous to the subconjunctival space.

of 26.3 to 14.3 mm Hg at 12 months and to 14.6 mm Hg in 16 patients at 24 months; moreover, 87.7% of the eyes had achieved an IOP below 18 mm Hg at 12 months.

Ultrasound

While minimally invasive approaches to glaucoma surgery have much improved safety profile, they all suffer from the fundamental, albeit minimized, risk of intraocular surgery and must be done in an operating room. In contrast, noninvasive approaches such as ultrasonic treatments are being developed for in-office use, targeting the same mild-to-moderate glaucoma population.[46] The concept is not new, as there has been evidence since the mid-1980s that ultrasonic energy can lower IOP.[47-50]

EyeTechCare (Rilleux-la-Pape, France) has developed a device called the EyeOP1 that uses high-intensity focused ultrasound to trigger hyperthermia in focal areas of the ciliary body, leading to reduced aqueous humor production and consequently to reduced IOP.[47] The device currently has Conformité Européene (CE) approval for treatment of refractory glaucoma but is not yet approved in the United States. EyeOP1 allows treatment of the entire circumference of the eye (Figure 12-3) in approximately 1 minute, so the procedure can be performed in the examination room on an outpatient basis. Unlike laser cytodestruction, the treatment has not been associated with post-procedure inflammation or transient increases in IOP. In a study of EyeOP1 used at 2 different ultrasound exposure durations in 12 eyes of 12 patients with refractory glaucoma and uncontrolled IOP, the treatment significantly reduced IOP. Three-second exposure produced a reduction from a mean preoperative IOP of 36 to 28 mm Hg at one day after treatment; IOP was maintained at 27 mm Hg after 6 months. Four-second exposure produced a reduction from a mean preoperative IOP of 41 to 27 mm Hg at one day after treatment; IOP was maintained at 23 mm Hg after 6 months. EyeTechCare is collecting data from additional patients throughout Europe to confirm the efficacy and positive safety profile of EyeOP1 and may seek approval for indications beyond refractory glaucoma if the evidence is supportive.

Another ultrasonic device, designed by cataract surgeon Donald Schwartz and currently under development at Eye Sonix (Long Beach, CA), targets increased aqueous humor outflow as the means of lowering IOP.[47] This is achieved by creating localized hyperthermia both at the TM and in the angle. After applying the device outside of the eye and adjacent to the limbus, ultrasound is delivered circumferentially around the limbus for several seconds. According to Dr. Schwartz, the

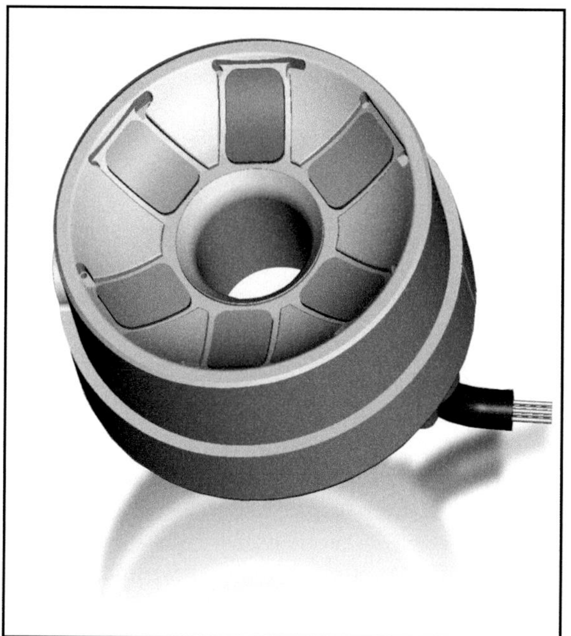

Figure 12-3. Ultrasound eye docking unit, which allows for 360-degree treatment of ciliary processes.

device increases temperature at the target area sufficient to trigger a cytokine cascade but insufficient to be painful or cause cell necrosis. Theoretically, the cytokine cascade leads to production of enzymes that break down TM debris and to induction of macrophages that clear the debris away, resulting in increased outflow through the TM. Initial unpublished clinical feasibility experience from the company purports an IOP-lowering effect comparable to that achieved with selective laser trabeculoplasty.

Deep Wave Trabeculoplasty

Deep wave trabeculoplasty (DWT) is an emerging therapeutic modality that leverages the use of focused mechanical oscillations over the TM, which then results in remodeling of the outflow system and lowering of IOP. The entire treatment is completed noninvasively along the tissues proximate to the limbus (Figure 12-4). Preclinical research has demonstrated that the cyclical stretch of the TM induced by the mechanical oscillations results in production of cytokines that could then lead to the observed decrease in IOP.[51,52] The initial preclinical testing involved brown Norway rats. Prior to initial treatment, the average IOP (mm Hg, SD) was 28.22 +/- 1.48 and 27.78 +/- 1.47 for the study and control eyes, respectively. The average initial IOP check 2 minutes after treatment was 26.67 +/- 1.80 for the treatment eyes and 27.67 +/- 1.49 for the control eyes. IOP check at 15 minutes revealed average pressures of 25.56 +/- 1.59 for the treated eyes and 27.33 +/- 1.05 for the control eyes. After one week, the treatment eyes had an average IOP of 21.56 +/- 1.13 and the control eyes had an average IOP of 27.89 +/- 0.99.[53] A follow-up study on New Zealand white rabbits showed treated eyes experienced a decrease in IOP (mm Hg, SD) from 16.13 +/- 1.46 to 12.25 +/- 2.31. This represented a 3.88 point (24%) decrease in IOP. In contrast, control eyes did not experience any significant decrease in IOP from baseline. In addition, the level of matrix metalloproteinase-2 (MMP2), implicated as having a role in the effect of laser trabeculoplasty on the TM, in the aqueous humor of treated rabbits increased significantly between pretreatment levels and week 1 levels. MMP2 staining increased and TIMP metallopeptidase inhibitor 2 staining remained stable in the TM of treated eyes compared to control eyes. These findings are similar to previously reported publications involving laser trabeculoplasty. There was

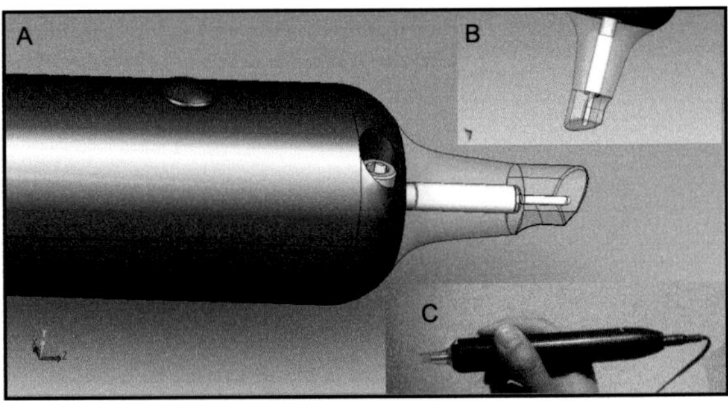

Figure 12-4. (A) The mechanical oscillator is fashioned with a distal tip that conforms to the limbal anatomy and features (B) an oscillating tip that depresses the tissue overlying the TM leading to repeated stretching of the tissue. (C) The device is manufactured to allow for a hand-held approach.

no evidence of trauma to the treated tissues. More recently, human studies were carried out and revealed safe and successful lowering of IOP for 3 months. Enrollment criteria included a diagnosis of OAG with wash out IOP > 23 mm Hg. Success of treatment was defined as a reduction in IOP of at least 20% and a decrease in medication use from baseline. Treated eye IOP decreased from a baseline washout of 24.27 to 17.87 mm Hg at 3 months. Average medication use in treated eyes also decreased from 2.0 prior to treatment to 0.3 medications in successfully treated eyes. Overall, 70% of treated eyes were classified as successful according to study criteria. These findings were significantly better than the IOP profile post-treatment in control eyes.

Wound Modulation

MIGS offers numerous advantages over conventional glaucoma surgeries by being anatomically precise, less traumatic, and safer. As discussed in this book, a variety of stent or shunt devices have been introduced for aqueous humor drainage. By targeting the physiological outflow pathways in the eye, the trabecular outflow or uveoscleral outflow system, these newer devices minimize or eliminate many complications encountered with standard incisional glaucoma surgeries. Although earlier studies on MIGS procedures appeared promising in terms of their efficacy and safety, prospective longitudinal clinical trials are warranted to compare their efficacy to established gold standards and to determine their role in the glaucoma surgical armamentarium.

As with conventional surgeries, concerns remain about late failures with these devices because of scar tissue formation. Obstruction of drainage channels within the Gold Micro-Shunt (SOLX Corp, Waltham, MA) has already been reported. Figus et al[54] reported the presence of a thin membrane that obstructed anterior holes of the Gold Micro-Shunt in 66.7% of failures. In another study, Agnifili et al[55] investigated the histological features of failed Gold Micro-Shunts and reported excessive connective tissue deposition and formation of a thick, fibrous capsule around both the proximal and distal tails of the shunt. Early pilot studies with the Aquashunt (Opko Health, Inc, Miami, FL) found fibrosis in the suprachoroidal space to be responsible for late surgical failures. These preliminary reports indicate that wound modulation may be required with these newer devices and will continue to be an active area of research to optimize surgical outcomes of glaucoma surgery.

Various alternatives for wound modulation are currently being used and investigated to reduce inflammation and late failures in conventional glaucoma surgeries. The 2 antimetabolites commonly used during trabeculectomy are mitomycin C (MMC) and 5-fluorouracil (5-FU). Although these drugs have been shown to significantly improve surgical outcomes, no standardized protocol currently exists for their use.[56-60] Moreover, higher rates of complications including bleb leaks, hypotony, and infection have been reported with their use.[58,61,62] Therefore, recent research has focused on amniotic membranes, antivascular endothelial growth factor agents, and tissue-engineered biodegradable implants to minimize complications observed with antimetabolites. The benefit of these newer approaches or their modifications for MIGS procedures, especially the ab externo techniques, remains to be tested, but their current use is briefly discussed next.

Amniotic membrane and antivascular endothelial growth factor (anti-VEGF) agents have been demonstrated to enhance bleb survival after trabeculectomy in animal models.[63,64] Subconjunctival use of anti-VEGF agents has reduced bleb vascularity with improved IOP control in various clinical studies.[65,66] Recently, Nilforushan et al[67] published their research with subconjunctival bevacizumab (2.5 mg/0.1 mL) versus MMC (0.02% for 3 min) in a randomized study of 36 eyes undergoing trabeculectomy. At 8 months follow-up, significant IOP reduction was noted in both groups; IOP was reduced from 21.9 ± 7.9 to 13.6 ± 3.2 mm Hg in the bevacizumab group and from 23.3 ± 4.9 to 9.6 ± 2.7 mm Hg in the mitomycin C group. No adjunctive glaucoma medications were required in the MMC group, whereas the bevacizumab group required 0.2 ± 0.5 medications.

Another recent development is the use of collagen matrix for wound modulation. Ologen collagen matrix implant (Optous, Roseville, CA) has been approved by the FDA for use during trabeculectomy. It is currently being investigated in a multicenter, prospective, randomized trial. This artificial porcine, extracellular matrix provides a scaffold for growth of fibroblasts and results in tissue remodeling and reduction of scar formation.[68,69] Eventually, the implant dissolves and results in a more physiologically appearing bleb that may reduce the risk of late complications of bleb leaks and infection seen with avascular, cystic blebs after current antimetabolite therapy.

Efficacy of Ologen collagen matrix implant has been demonstrated in both animal and human studies. In one randomized study comparing trabeculectomy alone versus trabeculectomy with Ologen, comparable IOP reduction was reported in both groups at 6 months without any difference in postoperative complications or adjunctive glaucoma medications.[70] In another prospective study comparing trabeculectomy outcomes with Ologen and MMC, comparable IOP reduction was reported in both groups at 12 months, with more eyes in the Ologen group requiring postoperative glaucoma medications.[71] In a prospective randomized trial evaluating the efficacy of Ologen implant or MMC as adjuvant agent in trabeculectomy, Cillino et al[72] demonstrated significant and comparable IOP reduction in both groups at 24 months. The investigators also assessed bleb elevation by using spectral domain optical coherence tomography and Moorfields Bleb Grading System. Bleb elevation was more pronounced in the Ologen group, and the imaging modality provided some differentiation between the functional and nonfunctional blebs.

From drug delivery to wound modulation, advances in the medical and surgical treatment of glaucoma are occurring at a rapid and exciting pace. We expect that future editions of this text will allow us to expand on the knowledge presented in this chapter.

References

1. Kompella UB, Kadam RS, Lee VH. Recent advances in ophthalmic drug delivery. *Ther Deliv.* 2010;1(3):435-56.
2. Gooch N, Molokhia SA, Condie R, et al. Ocular drug delivery for glaucoma management. *Pharmaceutics.* 2012;4:197-211.
3. QLT announces encouraging phase II data from CORE study of punctal plug drug delivery system. [news release]. Vancouver, Canada: QLT Inc; October 28, 2008. http://www.qltinc.com/newsCenter/2008/081028b.htm. Accessed October 2012.
4. Ocular Therapeutix Demonstrates Two-Month IOP Reduction with Sustained Release Travoprost for the Treatment of Glaucoma [news release]. Bedford, MA: Ocular Therapeutix, Inc; October 30, 2012. http://www.ocutx.com/us/2012/10/30/ocular-therapeutix-demonstrates-two-month-iop-reduction-with-sustained-release-travoprost-for-the-treatment-of-glaucoma/. Accessed October 2012.
5. Fezza JP, Gindoff S. Study raises concern over plug: The Medennium SMARTPlug may be associated with an increased incidence of canaliculitis. *Rev Ophthalmol.* March 21, 2011.
6. Schultz CL, Poling TR, Mint JO. A medical device/drug delivery system for treatment of glaucoma. *Clin Exp Optom.* 2009;92(4):343-348.
7. Kim J, Conway A, Chauhan A. Extended delivery of ophthalmic drugs by silicone hydrogel contact lenses. *Biomaterials.* 2008;29(14):2259-2269.
8. Gulsen D, Chauhan A. Ophthalmic drug delivery through contact lenses. *Invest Ophthalmol Vis Sci.* 2004;45(7):2342-7.

9. Gulsen D, Chauhan A. Dispersion of microemulsion drops in HEMA hydrogel: a potential ophthalmic drug delivery vehicle. *Int J Pharm.* 2005;292(1-2):95-117.
10. Gulsen D, Li CC, Chauhan A. Dispersion of DMPC liposomes in contact lenses for ophthalmic drug delivery. *Curr Eye Res.* 2005;30(12):1071-1080.
11. Kapoor Y, Thomas JC, Tan G, John VT, Chauhan A. Surfactant-laden soft contact lenses for extended delivery of ophthalmic drugs. *Biomaterials.* 2009;30(5):867-878.
12. Danion A, Brochu H, Martin Y, Vermette P. Fabrication and characterization of contact lenses bearing surface-immobilized layers of intact liposomes. *J Biomed Mater Res A.* 2007;82(1):41-51.
13. Danion A, Arsenault I, Vermette P. Antibacterial activity of contact lenses bearing surface-immobilized layers of intact liposomes loaded with levofloxacin. *J Pharm Sci.* 2007;96(9):2350-2363.
14. Ciolino JB, Hoare TR, Iwata NG, et al. A drug-eluting contact lens. *Invest Ophthalmol Vis Sci.* 2009;50(7):3346-3352.
15. Ghate D, Edelhauser HF. Barriers to glaucoma drug delivery. *J Glaucoma.* 2008;17(2):147-156.
16. Hiratani H, Alvarez-Lorenzo C. Timolol uptake and release by imprinted soft contact lenses made of N,N-diethylacrylamide and methacrylic acid. *J Control Release.* 2002;83(2):223-230.
17. Alvarez-Lorenzo C, Yanez F, Barreiro-Iglesias R, Concheiro A. Imprinted soft contact lenses as norfloxacin delivery systems. *J Control Release.* 2006;113(3):236-244.
18. Ali M, Horikawa S, Venkatesh S, Saha J, Hong JW, Byrne ME. Zero-order therapeutic release from imprinted hydrogel contact lenses within in vitro physiological ocular tear flow. *J Control Release.* 2007;124(3):154-162.
19. Witcherle O, Lim D. Hydrophilic gels for biological use. *Nature.* 1960;185:117-118.
20. Saati S, Lo R, Li PY, Meng E, Varma R, Humayun MS. Mini drug pump for ophthalmic use. *Curr Eye Res.* 2010;35:192-201.
21. University of Kentucky. Safety Study of Latanoprost Slow Release Insert (Latanoprost SR) [clinical trial NCT01180062]. http://clinicaltrials.gov/ct2/show/NCT01180062.
22. Patel SR, Lin ASP, Edelhauser HF, Prausnitz MR. Suprachoroidal drug delivery to the back of the eye using hollow microneedles. *Pharm Res.* 2011;28(1):166–176.
23. Patel SR, Berezovsky DE, McCarey BE, Zarnitsyn V, Edelhauser HF, Prausnitz MR. Targeted administration into the suprachoroidal space using a microneedle for drug delivery to the posterior segment of the eye. *Invest Ophthalmol Vis Sci.* 2012;53(8):4433-4441.
24. Patel SR, Berezovsky DE, McCarey BE, Zarnitsyn V, Edelhauser HF, Prausnitz MR. Targeted administration into the suprachoroidal space using a microneedle for drug delivery to the posterior segment of the eye. *Invest Ophthalmol Vis Sci.* 2012;53(8):4433-41.
25. Olsen TW, Feng X, Wabner K, Csaky K, Pambuccian S, Cameron JD. Pharmacokinetics of pars plana intravitreal injections versus microcannula suprachoroidal injections of bevacizumab in a porcine model. *Invest Ophthalmol Vis Sci.* 2011;52(7):4749-4756.
26. Olsen TW, Edelhauser HF, Lim JI, Geroski DH. Human scleral permeability. Effects of age, cryotherapy, transscleral diode laser, and surgical thinning. *Invest Ophthalmol Vis Sci.* 1995;36(9):1893-1903.
27. Olsen TW, Feng X, Wabner K, et al. Cannulation of the suprachoroidal space: a novel drug delivery methodology to the posterior segment. *Am J Ophthalmol.* 2006;142(5):777-787.
28. Augustin C, Augustin A, Tetz M, Rizzo S. Suprachoroidal drug delivery--a new approach for the treatment of severe macular diseases. *European Ophthalmic Review.* 2012;6:25-27.
29. Patel SR, Lin AS, Edelhauser HF, Prausnitz MR. Suprachoroidal drug delivery to the back of the eye using hollow microneedles. *Pharm Res.* 2011;28(1):166-176.
30. Peden MC, Min J, Meyers C, et al. Ab-externo AAV-mediated gene delivery to the suprachoroidal space using a 250 micron flexible microcatheter. *PLoS One.* 2011;6(2):e17140.
31. Ianchulev T, Rau MB, Khatana A, Craven E. Intraocular Pressure–Lowering Effect of Suprachoroidal Microstent in Combination With Phaco Cataract Surgery. Presented at American Academy of Ophthalmology annual meeting; November 2012; Chicago, IL.
32. American Academy of Ophthalmology. Primary open-angle glaucoma PPP - October 2010. http://one.aao.org/CE/PracticeGuidelines/PPP_Content.aspx?cid=93019a87-4649-4130-8f94-b6a9b19144d2. Accessed November 2012.
33. Mansouri K, Medeiros FA, Tafreshi A, Weinreb RN. Continuous 24-hour monitoring of intraocular pressure patterns with a contact lens sensor. *Arch Ophthalmol.* 2012;130(12):1534-1539.
34. Pinchuk L, Wilson GJ, Barry JJ, Schoephoerster RT, Parel JM, Kennedy JP. Medical applications of poly(styrene-block-isobutylene-block-styrene) ("SIBS"). *Biomaterials.* 2008;29(4):448-460.
35. Acosta AC, Espana EM, Yamamoto H, et al. A newly designed glaucoma drainage implant made of poly(styrene-b-isobutylene-b-styrene): biocompatibility and function in normal rabbit eyes. *Arch Ophthalmol.* 2006;124(12):1742-1749.
36. Wise JB, Witter SL. Argon laser therapy for open-angle glaucoma. A pilot study. *Arch Ophthalmol.* 1979;97(2):319-322.

37. Latina MA, Park C. Selective targeting of trabecular meshwork cells: in vitro studies of pulsed and CW laser interactions. *Exp Eye Res.* 1995;60(4):359-371.
38. Seibold LK, Kahook MY. Potential applications for femtosecond lasers in glaucoma. *Glaucoma Today.* 2012.
39. Nagy Z, Takacs A, Filkorn T, Sarayba M. Initial clinical evaluation of an intraocular femtosecond laser in cataract surgery. *J Refract Surg.* 2009;25(12):1053-1060.
40. Toyran S, Liu Y, Singha S, et al. Femtosecond laser photodisruption of human trabecular meshwork: an in vitro study. *Exp Eye Res.* 2005;81(3):298-305.
41. Nakamura H, Liu Y, Witt TE, Gordon RJ, Edward DP. Femtosecond laser photodisruption of primate trabecular meshwork: an ex vivo study. *Invest Ophthalmol Vis Sci.* 2009;50(3):1198-2104.
42. Bahar I, Kaiserman I, Trope GE, Rootman D. Non-penetrating deep sclerectomy for glaucoma surgery using the femtosecond laser: a laboratory model. *Br J Ophthalmol.* 2007;91(12):1713-1714.
43. Chai D, Chaudhary G, Mikula E, Sun H, Juhasz T. 3D finite element model of aqueous outflow to predict the effect of femtosecond laser created partial thickness drainage channels. *Lasers Surg Med.* 2008;40(30):188-195.
44. Chai D, Chaudhary G, Mikula E, Sun H, Kurtz R, Juhasz T. In vivo femtosecond laser subsurface scleral treatment in rabbit eyes. *Lasers Surg Med.* 2010;42(7):647-651.
45. Geffen N, Ton Y, Degani J, Assia EI. CO2 laser-assisted sclerectomy surgery, part II: multicenter clinical preliminary study. *J Glaucoma.* 2012;21(3):193-198.
46. Aptel F, Lafon C. Therapeutic applications of ultrasound in ophthalmology. *Int J Hyperthermia.* 2012;28(4):405-418.
47. Kent C. Using ultrasound to reduce high IOP. *Review of Ophthalmology.* 2012.
48. Valtot F, Kopel J, Haut J. Treatment of glaucoma with high intensity focused ultrasound. *Int Ophthalmol.* 1989;13(102):167-170.
49. Coleman DJ, Lizzi FL, Driller J, et al. Therapeutic ultrasound in the treatment of glaucoma. I. Experimental model. *Ophthalmology.* 1985;92(3):339-346.
50. Coleman DJ, Lizzi FL, Driller J, et al. Therapeutic ultrasound in the treatment of glaucoma. II. Clinical applications. *Ophthalmology.* 1985;92(3):347-353.
51. Bradley JM, Kelley MJ, Zhu X, Anderssohn AM, Alexander JP, Acott TS. Effects of mechanical stretching on trabecular matrix metalloproteinases. *Invest Ophthalmol Vis Sci.* 2001;42(7):1505-1513.
52. Ramos RF, Sumida GM, Stamer WD. Cyclic mechanical stress and trabecular meshwork cell contractility. *Invest Ophthalmol Vis Sci.* 2009;50(8):3826-3832.
53. Kahook MY, inventor; The Regents of the University of Colorado, a Body Corporate, assignee. A Non-Invasive Device for Lowering Intraocular Pressure. World patent WO 2009/155114. 2009 Dec 23.
54. Figus M, Lazzeri S, Fogagnolo P, Iester M, Martinelli P, Nardi M. Supraciliary shunt in refractory glaucoma. *Br J Ophthalmol.* 2011;95(11):1537-1541.
55. Agnifili L, Costagliola C, Figus M, et al. Histological findings of failed gold micro shunts in primary open-angle glaucoma. *Graefes Arch Clin Exp Ophthalmol.* 2012;250(1):143-149.
56. Singh K, Mehta K, Shaikh NM, et al. Trabeculectomy with intraoperative mitomycin C versus 5-fluorouracil. Prospective randomized clinical trial. *Ophthalmology.* 2000;107(12):2305-2309.
57. WuDunn D, Cantor LB, Palanca-Capistrano AM, et al. A prospective randomized trial comparing intraoperative 5-fluorouracil vs mitomycin C in primary trabeculectomy. *Am J Ophthalmol.* 2002;134(4):521-528.
58. Five-year follow-up of the Fluorouracil Filtering Surgery Study. The Fluorouracil Filtering Surgery Study Group. *Am J Ophthalmol.* 1996;121(4):349-366.
59. Rothman RF, Liebmann JM, Ritch R. Low-dose 5-fluorouracil trabeculectomy as initial surgery in uncomplicated glaucoma: long-term followup. *Ophthalmology.* 2000;107(6):1184-1190.
60. Sidoti PA, Choi JC, Morinelli EN, et al. Trabeculectomy with intraoperative 5-fluorouracil. *Ophthalmic Surg Lasers.* 1998;29(7):552-561.
61. Greenfield DS, Liebmann JM, Jee J, Ritch R. Late-onset bleb leaks after glaucoma filtering surgery. *Arch Ophthalmol.* 1998;116(4):443-447.
62. Soltau JB, Rothman RF, Budenz DL, et al. Risk factors for glaucoma filtering bleb infections. *Arch Ophthalmol.* 2000;118(3):338-342.
63. Wang L, Liu X, Zhang P, Lin J. An experimental trial of glaucoma filtering surgery with amniotic membrane [in Chinese]. *Yan Ke Xue Bao.* 2005;21(2):126-131.
64. Memarzadeh F, Varma R, Lin LT, et al. Postoperative use of bevacizumab as an antifibrotic agent in glaucoma filtration surgery in the rabbit. *Invest Ophthalmol Vis Sci.* 2009;50(7):3233-3237.
65. Kapetansky FM, Pappa KS, Krasnow MA. Subconjunctival injection(s) of bevacizumab for failing filtering blebs [E-Abstract 4149]. In: Association for Research in Vision and Ophthalmology; 2008; Ft. Lauderdale, FL: *Invest Ophthalmol Vis Sci*; 2008.
66. Purcell JM, Teng CC, Tello C. Effect of needle bleb revision with ranibizumab as a primary intervention in a failing bleb following trabeculectomy [E-Abstract 4165]. In: Association for Research in Vision and Ophthalmology; 2008; Ft. Lauderdale, FL: *Invest Ophthalmol Vis Sci*; 2008.

67. Nilforushan N, Yadgari M, Kish SK, Nassiri N. Subconjunctival bevacizumab versus mitomycin C adjunctive to trabeculectomy. *Am J Ophthalmol.* 2012;153(2):352-357.e1.
68. Chen HS, Ritch R, Krupin T, Hsu WC. Control of filtering bleb structure through tissue bioengineering: An animal model. *Invest Ophthalmol Vis Sci.* 2006;47(12):5310-5314.
69. Hsu WC, Ritch R, Krupin T, Chen HS. Tissue bioengineering for surgical bleb defects: an animal study. *Graefes Arch Clin Exp Ophthalmol.* 2008;246(5):709-717.
70. Papaconstantinou D, Georgalas I, Karmiris E, et al. Trabeculectomy with OloGen versus trabeculectomy for the treatment of glaucoma: a pilot study. *Acta Ophthalmol.* 2010;88(1):80-85.
71. Rosentreter A, Schild AM, Jordan JF, Krieglstein GK, Dietlein TS. A prospective randomised trial of trabeculectomy using mitomycin C vs an ologen implant in open angle glaucoma. *Eye (Lond).* 2010;24(9):1449-1457.
72. Cillino S, Di Pace F, Cillino G, Casuccio A. Biodegradable collagen matrix implant vs mitomycin-C as an adjuvant in trabeculectomy: a 24-month, randomized clinical trial. *Eye (Lond).* 2011;25(12):1598-1606.

Financial Disclosures

Dr. Iqbal Ike Ahmed consults for or receives consulting fees from Abbott Medical Optics, AdeTherapeutics, ACE Vision Group, Alcon, Allergan, AqueSys, Carl Zeiss Meditec, Clarity Medical Systems, EndoOptiks, Eyelight, ForSight Labs, Glaukos, InnFocus, Iridex, Ivantis, Liquidia Technologies, Inc, Ono Pharma, Sensimed, SOLX, Stroma, Transcend Medical, and TrueVision; receives speakers honoraria from Abbott Medical Optics, Alcon, Allergan, Carl Zeiss Meditec, Clarity Medical Systems, Mastel, MST Surgical, and Neomedix; and receives research grants/support from Abbott Medical Optics, Alcon, Allergan, AqueSys, Carl Zeiss Meditec, Glaukos, Ivantis, New World Medical, SOLX, and Transcend Medical.

Dr. John P. Berdahl has no financial or proprietary interest in the materials presented herein.

Dr. Jacob W. Brubaker has no financial or proprietary interest in the materials presented herein.

Dr. Sean Ianchulev is chief medical officer for Transcend Medical.

Dr. Sabita M. Ittoop has no financial or proprietary interest in the materials presented herein.

Dr. Malik Y. Kahook receives research grants from Alcon, Allergan, B&L, Regeneron, Genentech, ClarVista Medical, State of Colorado, and AMO; consults for Alcon, Allergan, ClarVista Medical, AMO, Valeant, and Aerie Pharma; and holds intellectual property for Glaukos, ClarVista Medical, ShapeOphthalmics, ShapeTech, Oasis, and AMO.

Dr. Ananda Kalevar has no financial or proprietary interest in the materials presented herein.

Dr. Mahmoud Khaimi has no financial or proprietary interest in the materials presented herein.

Dr. Mina B. Pantcheva has no financial or proprietary interest in the materials presented herein.

Dr. Hady Saheb has received travel funding from Glaukos, Ivantis Inc, and Transcend Medical.

Dr. Sarwat Salim is a lecturer for Alcon and Merck.

Dr. Thomas W. Samuelson is a consultant to AqueSys, Glaukos, and Ivantis.

Mr. Andrew Schieber is an employee of Ivantis.

Dr. Leonard K. Seibold receives research support/funding from Alcon and Sensimed.

Dr. Kuldev Singh is a consultant for Alcon, Allergan, Bausch and Lomb, Ivantis, and Transcend.

Dr. Jeffrey R. SooHoo has no financial or proprietary interest in the materials presented herein.

Dr. Carol B. Toris receives research support from Glaukos and Ivantis.

Dr. Rohit Varma is a consultant to Allergan, Inc, AqueSys, Genentech, Merck and Co, Inc, and Replenish and receives grants from Genentech, National Eye Institute, and Replenish, Inc.

Index